THE
SLIPPED DISC

James Cyriax MD (Cantab), MRCP (London)

Honorary Consulting Physician in Orthopaedic Medicine
St Thomas's Hospital, London

Visiting Physician in Orthopaedic Medicine
Rochester University Medical Centre, New York

Second edition

Gower Press

First published in Great Britain by Gower Press Limited
Epping, Essex
1970

Reprinted 1971

Second edition 1975

© James Cyriax 1970 and 1975

ISBN 0 7161 0142 4

Set in 11 on 13 point Times and printed by
Tonbridge Printers Ltd, Peach Hall Works,
Shipbourne Road, Tonbridge, Kent.

Contents

5

Illustrations

Figures

Plates

(Between pages 80 and 81)

Preface

Disc-lesions present a world-wide problem. At any one moment more fit people are disabled by a slipped disc than by any other illness. Though the condition is so common, there remains a great dearth of doctors able to use the knowledge already in existence to their patients' advantage. Little provision exists in any country in the world for coping with the medical aspect of orthopaedics. This does not apply to the surgical aspect; in consequence, the few cases of slipped disc that require operation receive prompt and expert attention. But on the whole the rest—the vast majority —get short shrift within the medical sphere. Patients' unsatisfied demand has created a void that lay manipulators have been happy to exploit. Understandably enough, patients who have wandered in vain from one hospital department to another sooner or later look outside orthodox medicine. Yielding to their friends' insistence, they end up with manipulators of various persuasions—often osteopaths, chiropractors or bonesetters.

Lay manipulators sometimes succeed, sometimes fail, much to their own and their clients' puzzlement; yet simple reasons are not far to seek. Not having followed the medical curriculum, they cannot be sure whether, in any one case, manipulation is required or not. It is a question of trial and awaiting events. Nevertheless, in spite of working at such a disadvantage, they are well known for their dramatic successes on a small proportion of their clients. Up to a point, this is a boon; but how much better if the same relief had been afforded originally on doctors' orders within the medical field.

What the patient does not realise when visiting a lay manipulator is that the burden of diagnosis has been transferred to himself. He decides that manipulation is what he needs, then looks for someone to do it. Even then, he stands only a small chance of finding a lay manipulator who has actually completed a course of recognised training. Moreover, many disc displacements do not respond to manipulation, but often do well on alternative treatments, did patient and manipulator but know it. The unhappy sufferer, ignorant of these possibilities and often frequenting those whose understanding is little greater than his own, flounders unenviably between respect for outworn tradition and cultists' enthusiasms.

This is the glum prospect facing the ordinary man with a slipped disc today. All patients and all doctors are aware of these facts; the problem is neither unrecognised nor new. And it has gone on long enough. Just a century ago, Sir James Paget gave a lecture in London deploring "Cases that Bonesetters Cure" and there has been little change since, although the way bonesetters' spinal treatments achieve their good results has now been scientifically explained. The search for sound advice based on anatomical fact still baffles the average sufferer. There are simply not enough orthopaedic physicians to go round.

There is nothing obscure about a slipped disc. After all, the different ways in which a loose fragment can move within a joint cavity are finite and the results must be—and indeed are—predictable and ascertainable. Lay manipulators' specious assertions have clouded the air, and no sufficient counter from doctors has been forthcoming. Prevention, what can happen to a disc at various spinal levels, what can be done and what is the likely outcome are seldom difficult to determine. This book sets out the whole problem in simple language and logical sequence. It offers rational solutions which, given determination and good will on all sides, can be implemented without delay.

James Cyriax

Acknowledgements

I am grateful to my colleague, R. Barbor, for contributing the account of sclerosing injections in Chapter 5.

My thanks are due to Messrs Baillière, Tindall for permission to reprint illustrations already published in my *Orthopaedic Medicine,* volume 1.

1

The Slipped Disc

Disc trouble is all but universal. Few people reach middle age without suffering at one time or another from a crick in the neck, pain (often called "fibrositis") in one shoulder blade, neuritis in the arm, pain at the back of the chest perhaps radiating round to the ribs in front, backache, lumbago, sacro-iliac strain or sciatica. Many perfectly healthy people have had several of these disorders; very few escape altogether. These symptoms are those commonly occurring with different types of slipped disc at different levels along the spinal column. Other disorders causing these pains exist, of course, but they provide only a small minority of all cases. They are in the doctor's mind when he carries out the examination that distinguishes ordinary disc trouble from other, rarer conditions.

It must be made clear from the outset that the term "slipped disc," though a useful compression, is, strictly speaking, inaccurate. The whole disc does not slip out like a penny from a slot; indeed, as long as it is structurally sound, it cannot move. It is only when a crack has developed as the result of injury or of years of wear and tear, and has led to the formation of a loose piece, that this small fragment can shift and cause so much recurrent trouble.

Historical survey

The slipped disc is no new disease; indeed, the symptoms,
duration and treatment were all described centuries ago. In
1444, the Paston Letters mention the long time that the disorder takes to subside: "a cyetica that letted him a great
while to ride." Later, the same Letters (1477) describe a
"scyetyka" keeping a patient in bed for almost four months
—not very different from the average period off work today.
In 1673, the Duke of Albany noticed that the pain in his
leg stopped him standing upright: "the fitt of the seatick . . .
not being able to writ myself." Here is the first description
of the lumbar deformity forced on a patient compelled to
hold his joint tilted to make room for the displacement.
Shakespeare associated pain in the back with pain spreading
down the limb. In a list of diseases in *Troilus and Cressida,*
"loads of gravel i' th' back" figures in the same sentence as
"sciaticas"—correctly in the plural as there is more than one
cause of pain radiating along the course of the sciatic nerve.
He also noted that highly placed people were not immune:
"Thou cold sciatica cripple our senators" (*Timon of Athens*);
and was first to describe bilateral root pain: "Which of your
hips has the more profound sciatica?" (*Measure for Measure*).
  Traditional medical treatment has not changed much; it
was then—and, alas, often is even now—warmth. In 1640 it
was: "some soft woollen cloth which will preserve from lum-
baginous pains" and in 1667 Sir Jonas Moore cured his
sciatica "by boyling his buttocks." By 1722 "a catskin tanned
with the fur on and layd upon the part" was preferred.
Sensible treatment seems to have begun with laymen; for
Lady Stanhope reported in 1813 on the relief of lumbago by
manipulation by bath attendants in Turkey. Sir James Paget
deplored doctors' neglect of manipulation in a lecture, reported in *The Lancet* (1868), entitled "Cases That Bonesetters Cure"; his words apply with equal force today.
No wonder Emerson (1860) could draw attention to the re-
fractoriness to treatment: "If you have headache or sciatica

or leprosy, I beseech you by all angels to hold your peace."

The doctors were far behind Shakespeare. Though Vesalius had described the appearance of the intervertebral disc in 1555, the first book on sciatica (1864) does not mention the disc as a possible cause. The first account of a post-mortem examination revealing a protruded disc appeared in 1857; confirmation was tardy, one further case being reported in 1898, three more in 1919 and a further two in 1929. Puncture of the intervertebral disc in rabbits had already been found to cause protrusion in 1895. Though the second book on sciatica was published in 1864 by Lassègue, the test for stretching the nerve that is known by his name all over the continent of Europe was not mentioned by him at all, but was first described by one of his pupils in 1881. Charcot, the famous French neurologist, described the characteristic spinal deformity in 1888.

However, it was not until 1934 that two American surgeons (Mixter and Barr) wrote the original paper describing cure of sciatica by removal of a protruded disc. Lumbago was not attributed to a disc-lesion till eleven years later (Cyriax, 1945). The first complete account of sciatica, with X-ray photographs showing indentation of contrast material by the bulging disc, was written by Glorieux of Bruges in 1937. It is remarkable that this disease, given a name centuries ago, should have remained an enigma for so long, though it gave rise both to clear signs of derangement at a lumbar joint (which was often held visibly sideways on) and to restricted mobility of a sciatic nerve root (limited straight-leg raising).

The cervical and lumbar curves

The human spine is divided into three areas: cervical (neck), thoracic (chest) and lumbar—see Figure 1:1. It is surprising that the spine, though a weight-bearing structure, is constructed in curves. Architecturally, a vertical line would have been expected. The neck and lumbar concavities are compensated for by a convexity at the back of the chest, the centre of gravity of the body thus remaining poised vertically above the ankles. These concavities occur where disc trouble is commonest—at the fifth and sixth cervical and the fourth and fifth lumbar levels (see Figure 1:1). In my view, they have been developed in order to mitigate as far as possible the ill effects of compression on the spinal discs. The result of these two curves is that the tilt on the joint surfaces at the weakest levels is such as to exert a forward pressure on the disc. As long as the concavity is maintained, the compression stress due to the weight of the body pushes the disc forwards, away from the dura mater and the nerve roots (see Figures 1:2 and 1:3). Moreover, during impact from above or below, the curves give a little, again with shock-absorbing effect.

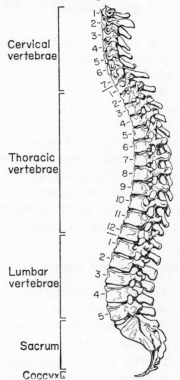

Cervical
vertebrae

Thoracic
vertebrae

Lumbar
vertebrae

Sacrum

Coccyx

FIGURE 1:1   THE THREE SPINAL CURVES

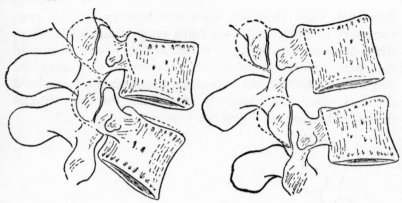

FIGURE 1:2 THE INCLINA-
TION OF THE LUMBAR JOINT
SURFACES WITH THE PATIENT
BENDING FULLY BACKWARDS

FIGURE 1:3 THE INCLINA-
TION OF THE LUMBAR JOINT
SURFACES WITH THE PATIENT
BENDING FULLY FORWARDS

Importance of correct posture

In the past, gymnastics and, even more, the health-and-beauty type of postural exercises have been based on aesthetic principles—that is, towards obliterating the normal spinal concavities at the neck and lower back. Unfortunately, this abolition produces the very posture most likely to set up disc trouble; it avoids the beneficial inclination of the joint surfaces that maintains the pressure pushing the disc away from the nerve roots. Hence, exercises involving bending down and touching the toes should be abandoned and children taught instead to keep their backs hollow, especially when lifting something heavy or sitting a long time. If this habit becomes ingrained and is continued into adult life, wanton straining of the back in the wrong direction will cease and each individual will keep his discs intact for as long as is possible.

A fetish exists that no one is "fit" unless he can bend and touch his toes. The ability to perform this feat is dependent upon the length of a person's hamstring muscles—that is, the muscles at the back of the thigh—and long ones are no better

B

than short ones. However, many people carry out this exercise every morning, and some bring on an attack of lumbago while doing so. It would be far better if they were to expend the same energy on using the back muscles to keep the lumbar spine hollow and then doing hands-on-hip, knees-bend exercises, since this selectively strengthens the very muscles that should be used in lifting (see Figure 1:4).

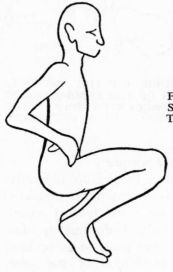

FIGURE 1:4 THE EXERCISE THAT SHOULD REPLACE BENDING TO TOUCH THE TOES: HANDS-ON-HIP, KNEES BEND

Anatomy

What is a slipped disc and why does it hurt?

Between the bodies of each two vertebrae lies a disc, except at the joint between the skull and the uppermost cervical vertebra, and the one below. There are thus twenty-four vertebrae and twenty-three discs.

The upper and lower surfaces of each vertebral body are covered by a thin shiny coating of gristle, exactly like that seen when carving a joint. Attached all the way round the edges of the bones, and to this layer of cartilage, is the disc. It lies between the bones and consists of a wide rim of cartilage surrounding a soft water-absorbent nucleus. The strips of cartilage are strong and arranged like the layers of an onion, with the fibres crossing at right angles for added strength. The nucleus distributes pressure hydrostatically—that is, equally in all directions—thus enabling the joint to bear considerable weight. But sooner or later cracks form and, since cartilage is a bloodless tissue, cannot heal. As long as the disc is intact, it cannot shift. Once it has cracked, the loose fragment is free to move (see Figure 1 : 5).

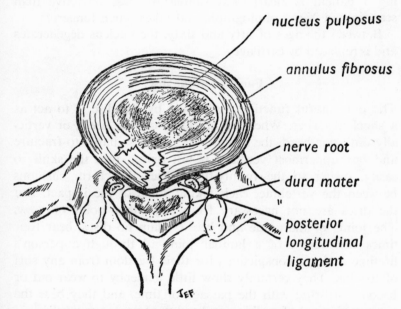

nucleus pulposus

annulus fibrosus

nerve root

dura mater

posterior longitudinal ligament

FIGURE 1:5 A CRACKED DISC (Front of body at top of figure)

It is this displacement that causes the trouble. The projection pinches sensitive structures, and pain in the trunk or limb results. The disorder has nothing to do with arthritis, any more than has a footballer's displaced cartilage in the knee. Moreover, a loose fragment may form and become displaced in a young person's spinal joint, normal on the X-ray photograph, or in an elderly patient's joint, when bony outcrops have already formed. Conversely, if degenerative changes exist without any disc displacement, no symptoms arise.

Since cartilage is a radio-translucent tissue, the ordinary X-ray photograph of the spinal joints cannot show whether or not a fragment of cartilage has moved. The best way— often the only way—to arrive at a correct diagnosis is by the evaluation of purely clinical criteria. In this assessment lies the root cause of much uncertainty, since examining a patient is clearly less simple and less objective than scanning an X-ray photograph, and takes much longer.

Between the ages of fifty and sixty, the nucleus degenerates and is replaced by cartilage.

Function of the disc

The only useful function performed by the disc is to act as a shock-absorber. When we fall erect on our heels, or vertically onto our head, the spinal bones are less liable to fracture and our uppermost vertebra is not driven into the skull so easily, owing to the twenty-three discs that form cushions between the vertebrae, each taking some of the impact. But the discs are not necessary from any other point of view. The joints of the ankle and heel contain no discs, bear four times the weight of a lumbar joint all through a person's lifetime and are conspicuous for their freedom from any sort of trouble. They certainly show little tendency to wear out or become arthritic with the passage of time, and they bear the repeated impact of walking on hard pavements very well.

Cause of pain

Originally, I had supposed by analogy that just as putting the cartilage out in a man's knee was known to make the blocked joint hurt, so would a displacement at a spinal joint set up pain also originating from the joint. This, however, proved false, for the mechanisms of pain at the knee and at the lumbar spine are different.

A number of clinical facts emerged during my studies that showed that a spinal joint was quite insensitive to displacement within itself. For example, there is a type of sciatica to which youngish people are prone, where the pain is felt in one limb only, never in the back at all. Yet the cause is a displaced disc at a low lumbar level. This and other clinical findings led me to the conclusion that the lumbar joint was insensitive to internal displacement; it was only when pressure was exerted on an adjacent sensitive structure that pain was experienced.

Lying behind the spinal joints is a central tube running down from the brain to the sacrum. The membrane contains the cerebro-spinal fluid in which the spinal cord floats and is called the dura mater. All the way down from the neck, pairs of spinal nerves emerge from the dura mater and pass through apertures between the vertebrae (the intervertebral foramina). Hence, centrally behind the joint lies the dura mater; just to each side lie the nerve roots. These are the two sensitive structures, impingement on which causes pain.

When a central backward displacement causes the ligament to bulge out enough to press it against the dura mater, pain in the centre of the neck, chest or back results, depending at which region of the spine the pressure is exerted (see Figure 1:6). If it passes to one side of the dura mater, the protrusion presses instead against the emergent nerve root (see Figure 1:7). Now, pain is felt in the territory supplied by that nerve root (arm, chest, abdomen or leg).

Usually, when the bulging fragment of disc shifts backwards to one side, it leaves the centre, thus liberating the dura mater. In consequence, as the pain in the upper limb, the front of the trunk or the lower limb comes on, the central pain normally ceases. By contrast, if a disc protrudes sideways or forwards, no sensitive structures lie close to these aspects of the joint, so that even large displacements in those directions cause no symptoms, though they give rise to remarkable bony spikes visible on the X-ray photograph (see Plate 3).

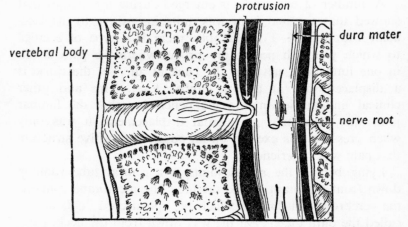

FIGURE 1:6 THE DISPLACEMENT IN LUMBAGO COMPRESSES
THE DURAL TUBE

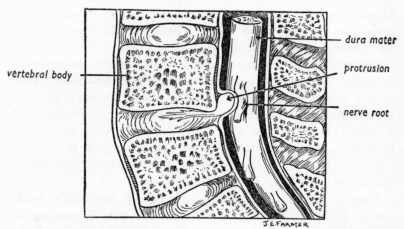

FIGURE 1:7 THE DISPLACEMENT IN SCIATICA COMPRESSES
THE NERVE ROOT

Frequency

The question may well be asked: why are disc-lesions so
common? A group of family doctors reported in 1966 that
in one year no less than one patient in forty on their list had
suffered pain severely enough to seek their advice. This takes

no account of patients with pain of spinal origin in the neck or chest, nor of those who suffered in silence, never bothering their doctor at all.

How is it that everyone can use his arms and legs for a lifetime with little liability to trouble, whereas exertion involving the spinal joints soon leads to pain and disablement? It must not be thought that the answer is merely a question of old age and inevitable degeneration. My youngest patient so far with a disc out in his neck was four years old; with lumbago, six years old. An orthopaedic colleague of mine swears that he had a little boy eighteen months of age walking in with his hand behind his back in the typical position of the old man in Figure 1:8. My earliest case of sciatica was a girl of eleven.

Relationship with evolutionary changes

Throughout the ages, the organs of the body have been altering continuously, evolving according to changes in function. For example, fishes' fins became lizards' legs when the capacity to breathe with lungs instead of gills became established. Monkeys' forelegs changed to arms when the body could be balanced upright; monkeys' nether hands ceased to be grasping mechanisms and became feet, adapting themselves to weight-bearing as the human race emerged. This is exactly what did *not* happen to the lumbar spine. This was originally a length-maintaining mechanism, connecting the pelvis and chest, leaving room for the abdomen. It was subject to extension strains—that is, backward, as, for example, when a horse is mounted by a rider—and learnt to bear them well. No proper provision was made for withstanding flexion strains— that is, bending forward—since a quadruped cannot bend forward: his forefeet are already on the ground. No proper provision was made for any compression stresses, since the lumbar spine, being slung horizontally, had never hitherto borne the weight of the body.

As soon as the development of the hind-brain became advanced enough to enable man to stand upright on two

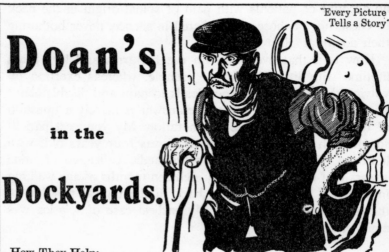

"Every Picture Tells a Story"

Doan's

in the

Dockyards.

How They Help:

Dockyards, workshops, mines and factories are more busy than ever before. Men and Women are working day and night. No one ever worked so hard.

It is no wonder the kidneys weaken, and backache, urinary disorder, gravel and rheumatic twinges result. For the kidneys' task is doubled by these days of strenuous body-racking work.

Doan's Backache Kidney Pills help by strengthening the work-worn kidneys. They help to purify the blood and to dislodge harmful uric-acid crystals.

Workers everywhere use Doan's Pills.

Read what loyal Dockyard Workers say:

Pembroke

A Six Year's Cure of a Very Bad Back. "Dockyard work is very hard, and a very bad back once made my work a burden.

Mr. J. Picton, 13 Imble Street, Bufferland, Pembroke Dock, gave this reminiscence on 3rd May, 1909, when he said:— "My kidney trouble was due to strain. It affected my back and caused bladder disorder and burning urination. I almost gave up work.

"Hearing at last of Doan's Pills, I followed the treatment. It cured me so thoroughly that I am now in first rate health. (Signed) J. PICTON."

Six Years' Proof. On October 16th, 1915, 6 years later, Mr. Picton said: "I am first-rate now, thanks to Doan's Pills. A good thing too, for there's plenty of work to do!"

Portsmouth

Lumbago after a Chill. 5 Years Cured. There is much to learn from the following dockyard experience. On September 20th, 1910, Mr. A. E. Allen of 218, Eastfield Road, Portsmouth, said:— "Lumbago after a chill once kept me from work for days. Sharp, stabbing backache used to take my breath away. I got quite weak from pain. Sediment indicated weak kidneys.

"Nothing did good except Doan's Pills. This medicine cured me absolutely. I haven't a sign of kidney trouble now. (Signed) A. E. Allen."

5 Years' Proof. On September 11th, 1915, Mr. Allen said:— "Doan's Pills so thoroughly rid me of lumbago and bladder trouble five years ago, that I have kept well ever since."

When You enter a Shop to Buy Doan's Pills

It is not enough to ask for kidney pills or backache pills. Ask distinctly for DOAN'S BACKACHE KIDNEY PILLS and be sure you get DOAN'S, like Mr. Picton and Mr. Allen had.

DOAN'S

Backache   Kidney   Pills.

All dealers or 2/9 a box from Foster McClellan Co. 8, Wells St. Oxford St. London W.

FIGURE 1:8   THE WELL-KNOWN ADVERTISEMENT FOR DOAN'S PILLS, SHOWING THE CHARACTERISTIC POSTURE IN LUMBAGO legs—and, biologically speaking, this is very recent—the function of the lower back became reversed. Now, for the first time, it was subjected to flexion and compression strains, neither of which it had ever been constructed to withstand. Though structures could still adapt themselves slightly, evolution had gone too far for a radical alteration in shape still to be possible. It was too late for the vertebral column to turn itself round through 180 degrees and face back to front. Man was, therefore, confronted not with a minor alteration but with a reversal of function, such as has not been required of any other tissue. The result was a basically unsound mechanism.

Not only that, but, by a piece of ill-fortune, at each level the sensitive spinal nerve root emerged opposite the joint containing the disc. In quadrupeds, the fact that the nerve lay opposite the weak joint did not matter, though it was fundamentally a piece of bad engineering. But in the human, whose disc was subject to compression with displacement, this poor design had unfortunate results. The course of the nerve should have been altered so that it left the spine by an aperture placed half way along the vertebral body. Then the disc could not have compressed the nerve root, however far it protruded backwards or sideways.

A quadruped's backbone requires strength to withstand extension strains; for example, a horse's spine must not break when the weight of a rider bends it backwards. In the course of evolution, therefore, a thick ligament was provided running along the front of the spine the whole way, and spanning the full width of each vertebral body. But the animal's spine never had to bear comparable flexion stress. Hence, no commensurately thick ligament was brought into being to ensure stability in flexion. Since the lumbar ligament running along the back of each joint had never had an important function, it was not only weaker, but at its lumbar extent did not even span the full width of the vertebra (see Figure 1:5). As a result, when a damaged disc protruded backwards a few times and met the central ligamentous resistance offered there, it tended to burrow to one or other side of the ligament, where there was no impediment. This event is signalled by disappearance of the backache and the substitution of pain down the leg—lumbago becoming sciatica. At the neck the names are different, the event being described as "fibrositis turning into neuritis," but the mechanism is the same.

Relationship to work

It was thought for many years, reasonably enough, that the heavier a man's work the more likely he would be to develop spinal trouble, especially in the lower back. This was found not to be so by Hult (1954), a surgeon working in northern Sweden, who looked after thousands of employees of a forestry company. He was, therefore, admirably placed to compare the incidence of lumbago in clerks and in tree-fellers and handlers. There was no difference in the frequency of attacks. The difference lay in the time that each individual had to stay off work. Sedentary employment enabled a man to hobble back to the office when only half-recovered, whereas the foresters had to wait till they were quite well again. Surprisingly enough, therefore, the executive travelling to the office by car and then seated, probably in an over-comfortable armchair, for most of the day is no less liable to back troubles than is his own gardener. It has since been shown that British dockers behave differently from Scandinavian foresters; for over here the dockers' rate for lumbago is ten times the national average.

Reason for the increase in disc trouble

The question is also often asked: surely disc trouble is becoming more frequent? Alternatively, is it just that the name has changed? The ascription *has* changed, of course; both lumbago and sciatica were once thought to be "rheumatism." But are they becoming more common? I am sure that they are. There is a consensus amongst elderly doctors that far more people suffer spinal trouble now than ever used to. It is true, of course, that more patients nowadays visit a doctor for complaints that they might well have suffered in silence in a more resigned age. Nevertheless, at the very moment when work is becoming less and less arduous everywhere in this country—indeed, heavy work in many trades has almost ceased—back trouble is becoming commoner. As far as the lower back goes, I attribute this to our sitting so much more than formerly.

A Swedish research-worker (Nachemson, 1959) inserted needles into the discs of patients while they lay, stood and sat, and took manometric readings. He found the pressure within the disc much the greatest when the individual sat. Whereas we used to walk everywhere, stood in the presence of our betters and sat very upright at meals, keeping the back hollow, we now slouch in armchairs, cars and aeroplanes, the back rounded for long periods at a time. As a result, the disc is subjected to continuous centrifugal pressure at the very time when the back is held convex. This posture entails the very tilt on the joint surfaces that forces the disc backwards towards the sensitive nervous tissues. This is the first time in history that man has spent much time sitting—the worst posture to adopt from the point of view of the disc.

Age factor

Back troubles are commonest in middle age, but I found during an investigation in 1944 that of my students, none of whom was over twenty years old, no less than one in four developed lumbar pain badly enough to come to see me in the course of three years' training.

Between the ages of fifty and sixty, the lumbar joints tend to stiffen slightly, and the movement to the full range that would have produced the displacement is no longer possible; hence, the tendency to lumbago often abates during that decade. During these years, bony outcrops are apt to form, especially at the mid-neck and the fourth and fifth lumbar joints. This condition is often called "osteoarthritis." By analogy with other joints, notably the hip, where degenerative changes do lead to pain, spinal osteoarthritis is often thought to cause symptoms. This is not so; in fact, the situation is reversed. The osteophytic outcrops cup the disc in bone, instead of softer ligaments, resulting in less movement. Osteoarthritis of the lumbar spine is, therefore, a beneficient phenomenon leading to greater stability of the joint and less likelihood of the fragment of disc shifting. When patients are told that their disc is degenerate and spinal osteoarthritis has set in, it must be indicated that this is not a painful condition; rather is it a cause for congratulation. Much apprehension is often needlessly aroused when, as the result of inspection of an X-ray film, words are used without due explanation. In the case in point, they have a wide and harmless connotation; the patient, complaining of discomfort, should be reassured that the bony outcrops, which have been present at the spine for years, cannot account for a recent condition. Moreover, they will still be there after he is quite well again.

Statistics from several countries show that disc troubles are commonest in middle age, rising to a peak between the ages of 50 and 60. Hence it is idle to maintain that disc degeneration and the formation of bony spikes are the cause of backache. Were this so, lumbar spinal troubles would inevitably get worse and more frequent as age advanced—the opposite of what actually happens. In fact, in really old people, backache is quite rare, in spite of increased degeneration.

Reason for recurrence

The discs consist largely of cartilage—an outer ring surrounding the water-absorbent nucleus. The only tissue in the body devoid of blood is cartilage. If a bone is broken or the skin is cut, blood is present and healing proceeds by the formation of new blood-borne tissue which bridges the breach. Cartilage lacks this power to unite; for, whatever the extent of the contact between the two broken surfaces of cartilage, nothing can form between them to heal them together. This is well known from cases where the meniscus has become torn in a footballer's knee; the loose piece stays loose, displacing itself again when the joint is used hard, causing such repeated annoyance that the cartilage has to be removed.

This is what also happens at a spinal joint. The loose fragment becomes displaced. It may go back into position by itself, or be reduced by manipulation or traction; it may slowly edge into position during relief from compression—in the case of lumbago, rest in bed. But the loose fragment stays loose, and the same exertion is followed, sooner or later, by another displacement. And so on. During my days as a medical student, when the broken cartilage had been put back in a patient's knee, some surgeons advocated resting the knee in plaster for some weeks in order to allow the crack to unite. Of course, this is now realised to be futile. No matter how long the joint is immobilised, a crack in cartilage cannot heal. In the absence of blood, whence can the uniting substance be derived? Nevertheless, plaster casts, though abandoned for the knee, are still sometimes prescribed for disc trouble with the stated, but vain, intention of letting the disc heal.

2

Symptoms and Signs of a Disc-Lesion

Disc troubles in the neck, in the thoracic extent of the spine and in the lumbar region behave rather differently from each other, and therefore merit separate consideration. Each spinal joint, except the two uppermost, contains a disc (see Figure 1:1). The common sites for a disc disorder are the lower cervical and the lower lumbar levels.

"Fibrositis"
Twenty-five years ago, an article in the *British Medical Journal* debunked "fibrositis," pointing out that the pain was genuine enough, but was not the result of an inflamed patch of fibrous tissue (Cyriax, 1948). On the contrary, it was a secondary phenomenon and owed its presence to a small disc displacement backwards. The pain was felt in the wrong place—that is, was referred—and was accompanied by an even more misleading tender spot which, when touched, was identified by the patient as the very source of his pain. But he was mistaken; the pain and tenderness were there, but were secondary to the primary joint lesion.

This faulty ascription led to endless trouble; for physiotherapists were asked to give heat and massage to painful but in fact normal tissues; or the doctor himself might inject a local anaesthetic solution there, or, more recently, hydrocortisone—all to no avail. Lay manipulators, so the patients found, could abolish the pain and tender spot by restoring painless movement to the spinal joint. After each successful shift of the loose fragment in the correct direction, the tender spot would alter its position, moving upwards and towards the centre of the lower neck as the displacement got less. This instant shift of the tender spot from place to place is one way of proving that it is not a patch of muscular inflammation. Another way is to test the muscle by making it contract strongly against resistance; this also shows that the muscle thought to be affected functions perfectly and painlessly. The trouble must, therefore, lie elsewhere.

Cervical disc-lesions

These go through seven stages, which are set out below. Only in the first three is the principal pain in the region of the neck. Most people never get beyond the second stage. Only a few individuals reach the final stage.

Acute torticollis

The first stage of cervical disc trouble goes by this name. The patient is young, aged somewhere between fifteen and thirty, and goes to bed feeling quite normal. Next morning he wakes and finds that he cannot lift his head off the pillow because of pain radiating from one ear down to the upper shoulder-blade area. This is the result of lying too still, for too long, on a pillow too thick or too thin. It usually happens on a Sunday morning. The patient is away for the weekend, staying with friends or at an hotel, and has been given a pillow of the wrong height for him. Moreover, there was a party and he drank too much. He therefore sleeps unduly soundly, without changing his posture in the ordinary way from time to time. As a result of keeping the neck sideways-on in one direction all night, the loose fragment of disc shifts its position and jams the joint. Consequently, the moment he first moves after waking he gets severe pain and finds that he has got a crick in his neck, which he can scarcely move. He avers that he must have been sleeping in a draught or that the innkeeper has not aired the sheets properly! For the first two or three days the pain is quite bad, constant, increased by moving the head and interferes with sleep. The attack subsides of its own accord and the whole episode has ceased in ten days. But it may occur again.

Examination shows that the head is held so that it is inclined to one side, in the position that affords the best relief—that is, in a manner which squeezes the displaced fragment the least—usually away from the painful side. When the movements of the neck are tested, bending forwards, backwards, sideways one way and turning one way may or may not hurt slightly, but there is no restriction. However, side-bending the other way and turning in that direction both prove impossible because of severe pain felt at one side of the neck. This blocking of the joint in two directions, but not in the other four, by a displaced chunk of disc has its parallel in the lumbar disc-lesion, in which the same type of partial painful restriction is often encountered.

Whiplash. Another way of developing acute torticollis is a whiplash injury. The patient is sitting in a stationary car which is run into from behind. The impact is unforeseen and the occupant cannot brace his muscles against it. The head is thrown backwards, then equally abruptly forwards, the unprotected joints bearing the brunt. Severe types of damage may be caused—even death—but the common result is a disc displacement, developing in the course of some hours, so that, by evening, pain prevents the neck being moved at all. Severe stiffness, sometimes with discomfort in both arms and pins and needles in the fingers, continues for several weeks, then slowly abates. Full movement returns after many months, but some degree of discomfort in the neck may remain, sometimes permanently. Unless the patient is claiming damages (when there is a tendency for symptoms to be prolonged until the suit is concluded some years later) the pain usually goes in the end, but genuine persistent symptoms, often relievable, are encountered.

Scapular pain

This second stage in cervical disc trouble was, during the early part of this century, miscalled "scapular fibrositis."

The patient is twenty to sixty years of age and finds himself subject to bouts of pain at one shoulder-blade, radiating perhaps up to the base of the skull. These attacks recur at intervals, say, once or twice a year (not necessarily on the same side each time), and while they last they make the neck stiff.

Examination shows that certain, but not all, movements of the neck evoke or increase the pain in the shoulder-blade area. It also shows that the trouble does not originate in the muscles at the shoulder-blade or neck; for, though a spot in one muscle is tender, testing it by a strong contraction against resistance is painless. These findings are charac-teristic of a block in part of a cervical joint, giving rise to pain felt on one side (as the loose fragment cannot move in both directions at once), increased on moving the joint. The displaced fragment is not so large and jams the joint less obviously than in acute torticollis, but they are both variants of the same condition.

"Brachial neuritis"

It is in the third stage of cervical disc trouble that pressure can be exerted on the nerve root as it emerges from the spine to run down the arm. The label, "brachial neuritis," is a bad one; for the lesion lies in the neck, not the arm (it is only the resulting pain that is felt in the arm—that is, brachial pain). Nor is it a neuritis, which is inflammation or degeneration of the conducting core of the nerve; for the nerve root is compressed from without and any interference with conduction is due to an extrinsic agency—that is, impact from the protruded disc (see Figure 2:1).

The patient is aged thirty-five to sixty and states that after

C

a bout of a week or two of accustomed pain in one shoulder-blade, just when subsidence was expected, the pain got worse and travelled down the arm to the hand, often causing pins and needles in some of the digits as well. The pain becomes increasingly severe for some weeks, then remains bad for another four to six weeks, is worse at night and prevents sleep. It then slowly abates. At the end of three to four months from the onset of the pain down the arm, the symptoms have ceased spontaneously. A second attack is most uncommon. (See Plate 2.)

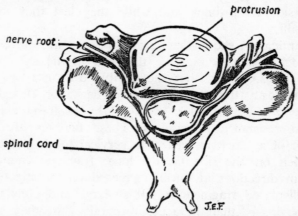

FIGURE 2:1   CERVICAL DISC COMPRESSING THE NERVE ROOT
(Front of body at top of figure)

Examination shows that some of the neck movements hurt in one shoulder-blade, exactly as they would have done before the pain spread down the upper limb. Only seldom does any movement of the neck project pain down the arm; if so, this is one of the signs that manipulation is likely to fail. The question now is: how large is the displacement? Is it large enough to squeeze the nerve root so hard that the group of muscles supplied by that root has lost strength? If so, manipulation is useless, but spontaneous recovery is almost certain to occur in three to four months (counting from when the pain in the *arm* started, not the pain at the shoulder-blade). If there is no weakness, manipulation may succeed, but not with the same ease as it would if the pain were confined to the shoulder-blade.

Once the pain has gone, the muscles recover their strength in the course of the next few months. Pressure of a protruded disc on a nerve root is a very disagreeable condition, but should not cause despair; for it does recover fully in the long run, without treatment.

An extremely annoying situation arises in connection with this disorder. After a few days of arm ache, the pain becomes such that the patient consults his doctor, who gives him analgesic tablets. At this point in time, the disorder is evolving; hence the patient reports a week later, at his second attendance, that he is worse. Stronger pills are ordered, again in vain. At his third attendance the patient is referred to a hospital. There he is X-rayed and told that he has a slipped disc in his neck, pressing on a nerve root, with weakened muscles in consequence. An electrical test on these muscles may be ordered and will confirm this finding. He may now be supplied with a collar, given traction or physiotherapy, none of which helps at all. By now the aggravation has ceased, but the constant pain interfering with sleep is very wearing.

After attending his doctor for several weeks and then hospital for, say, another month without getting any better, the patient despairs. He knows that he has a displaced disc pinching a nerve root; the hospital clearly cannot shift it. He, therefore, says to himself, logically enough, that he will suffer this pain for the rest of his life. This is entirely understandable, but is in fact untrue; spontaneous recovery is a virtual certainty. In desperation he now decides to go to a lay manipulator, at the very moment when recovery is about to start. He is treated, perhaps twice a week, on about twelve occasions—and gets well at exactly the same speed as if no treatment had been given. The cure has no connection with what has been done, but is related to the passage of six weeks. All "treatment" begun at the end of two months is sure to appear effective, but in reality no measure can even hasten spontaneous recovery. However, it is comprehensible why both the patient and the lay manipulator may imagine that the benefit resulted from the manipulations. How is either to know what is the natural history of this common disorder?

All that need be done, when an intractable displacement of this type is encountered, is to explain to the patient the chronological sequence that this disorder follows and to keep him under observation and adequately sedated until he is well.

Acroparaesthesia

This, the fourth stage, has no popular name. An elderly patient complains of vague aching up and down both arms, with the pins and needles in all five fingers of both hands. These symptoms come and go in an irregular way, day or night, never lasting long. (This transient behaviour must not be confused with the pins and needles felt in both hands which wake a middle-aged woman in the small hours each night, for this is unconnected with disc trouble.)

The cause is a bulge on the disc at each side of the joint, which is exerting slight pressure on one pair of emergent nerve roots. Later, the displacements may be replaced by bony outcrops.

Fifth, sixth and seventh stages

Few cases ever reach these late stages at all. A central bulge may slowly form and compress the dura mater. In consequence, central neckache, spreading to both shoulders, appears. If this displacement becomes larger, the spinal cord may be touched, causing pins and needles in feet and hands. Still further protrusion is a rarity, but when it occurs, it sets up sufficient pressure on the cord to make the legs weak.

Thoracic disc-lesions

Trouble with the discs at the joints that lie at the back of the chest is less common than at the neck and lower back, since the presence of ribs and of the breastbone restricts mobility. Moreover, the discs are thinner in relation to the size of the joint, and therefore allow less movement.

Thoracic backache

This is often the result of sitting slightly bent forwards all day—for example, when typing. By afternoon the upper back aches; getting up and standing straight, or walking about, brings relief in a few minutes. The pain is usually central or just to one side below the shoulder-blade.

Thoracic lumbago

A severe pain may come on suddenly, often while twisting the trunk during heavy lifting. If so, the patient is fixed in the manner of lumbago; he can scarcely move. The pain may radiate round the lower ribs towards the front of the chest on one or both sides. The patient has to take shallow breaths because deep expiration hurts, as does a cough.

Pain at the front of the trunk

Nearly all pains felt at the abdomen or the front of the chest are caused by internal trouble. Pain felt here because of pressure on a thoracic nerve root by a displaced fragment of disc does occur, however, and, since it may provoke no pain at all at the back of the chest, may give rise to considerable difficulties in diagnosis. The main distinction is, of course, that the pain is affected by posture, movement and exertion rather than by visceral function, such as eating.

It so happens that a case of this type may well be exhaustively investigated for internal trouble without any cause for the symptoms being detected. In consequence, the pain may be loosely attributed to some vague entity and the term "gastritis," or some such word, used. Should the patient now visit a lay manipulator, he may feel a click in his back and find his pain gone. The patient and the manipulator may thereupon decide that spinal manipulation cures gastritis, whereas, in fact, it cures only those thoracic displacements that have been mistaken for gastritis.

Examination

Whichever of these three types of disorder is present, the signs follow the standard pattern. Since a displacement exists at a spinal joint, blocking part of it, some movements hurt, others do not. The patient therefore bends forwards, backwards, to each side and then twists each way, reporting what he feels. In addition, the backward bulge may restrict the mobility of the dura mater or the nerve root. Hence, stretching these structures, by bending the head forwards or bringing the shoulder-blades backwards hard, may increase the pain in the trunk. Signs of impaired conduction along a thoracic nerve root or the spinal cord are rarely encountered.

Lumbar disc-lesions

These cause three different sets of symptoms and signs: backache, lumbago and sciatica. Each is considered separately.

Backache

Backache, central or just to one side of the lower back, coming on if the individual exerts himself and easing if he takes things quietly, is almost universal. There are two types of disc-lesion responsible for this condition: the hard and the soft.

The *hard* type of disc-lesion occurs when a loose piece of cartilage protrudes very slightly and then recedes again. An activity such as gardening may bring on some hours or days of pain, but a few days' respite brings complete relief. The *soft* type occurs when a small knuckle of nucleus bulges backwards after the joint has been held for a long time in the flexed position. In a case of this nature, the patient reports that after sitting for longer than, say, an hour—for example, when driving a car—his back begins to ache more and more, but that standing up straight stops the pain in a few minutes.

In either type, after months or years, the ache comes on

more readily, lasts longer and is more severe. In the end, it may last for months on end or even become permanent, because of a constant displacement.

Many women describe having had backache ever since a confinement. The cause of the backache is not the pregnancy, except that the circumstance provides the principal reason why a healthy woman might lie in bed for ten days in a faulty position (see Figures 6:10 and 6:11). It is the fact of having lain propped up in bed with a pillow at the back of the chest, but no support for the lower back, which, as a result, droops into convexity all day. Lying with the lower back flexed is no different from standing bent for a long time, but the patient is puzzled at backache coming on during a period of rest in bed, since she thinks that straining the back occurs as a result of heavy work.

At examination, the patient is asked to stand, whereupon the four movements of the lumbar spine are tested: bending forwards, backwards and to each side. Since the displacement blocks only part of the joint, all four movements seldom hurt. Usually, two or three hurt, the other one or two remaining free. There is also a curious sign present in early disc trouble that affords additional information—pain halfway down. The patient bends and, when he is halfway forwards, can be seen to falter momentarily, because of a pain that disappears as soon as he bends further forwards (see Figure 2:2). This sign indicates that there is something loose within the joint, which moves sharply when the tilt on the joint becomes reversed as flexion proceeds. Tests for impaired mobility of a nerve root and for lack of conduction prove negative. In other words, the signs relate to the affected lumbar joint only; everything else is normal.

Lumbago
Cartilaginous displacement. This is the result of the sudden appearance of a much larger displacement of disc substance (see Figure 1:6). The patient reports that he bent forwards to lift a weight and felt a sudden stab at the lower back, just

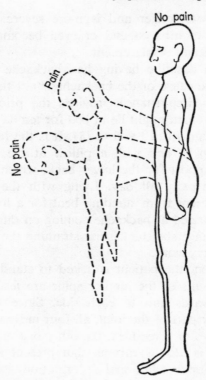

No pain

Pain

No pain

FIGURE 2:2 A PAINFUL ARC ON TRUNK FLEXION

at the beginning of the upward movement. He dropped the
weight and then found himself fixed bent forwards—occasionally bent sideways—because of severe pain on attempting
to achieve the upright position. He hobbles to bed and has to
lie there for several weeks until at last he is straight and getting up proves merely uncomfortable. At first, a cough hurts
at the lower back, and an unguarded movement, especially
turning in bed, occasions a severe twinge. Recovery is complete in the end, but he finds that, as from the first attack,
his back is never so strong again and exertion in the bent
position is apt to bring about an identical recurrence.

The signs are now very obvious. Since such a major displacement jams the lumbar joint severely, marked signs of

interference with mobility are to be expected. These are (*a*) *visible deformity*: the joint can be seen to be held in the position that best accommodates the displacement—bent forwards (see Plate 1) or bent sideways; (*b*) *limited movement*: some movements cannot be carried out at all whilst others are of full range, though not necessarily devoid of discomfort. In an extreme case, the patient may be able to bend sideways fully one way, whereas he cannot reach even the vertical position when he tries to bend the other way. In such cases the X-ray photograph shows two vertebrae held in angulation to make room for the displacement lying between them. This can be inferred, not actually seen; for the disc consists of cartilage—a radio-translucent tissue.

In ordinary backache the displacement is not large enough to cause clinical signs of interference with the mobility of the dura mater. But in lumbago, this phenomenon appears. Added to the signs of joint trouble, there is now (*c*) *pain on coughing*: a cough dilates the veins on the inner aspect of the dural tube, causing a momentary rise in the cerebro-spinal fluid pressure—this is transmitted in all directions, including downwards to the lumbar extent of the membrane, where it is jerked against the protrusion, causing pain; (*d*) *pain on stretching the dura mater*: when its mobility is impaired, the dural tube naturally resents being stretched. Hence bending the head forwards, stretching it from above, often hurts the lower back. Straight-leg raising while the patient lies on his back provides another method of stretching the dura mater, this time from below by way of each sciatic nerve. This movement is therefore very restricted and, since the protrusion lies centrally, neither leg can be lifted far during the first few days.

As the displacement recedes, whether slowly during recumbency or swiftly during manipulation, the first sign of improvement is an increased range of straight-leg raising. Later on, the fixation with visible spinal deformity gradually abates. Finally, one by one, the lumbar movements stop hurting, the last to do so usually being bending forwards.

Recovery is now complete. However, the crack in the disc that made the displacement possible in the first place cannot heal. Therefore, sooner or later, another similar strain will precipitate a further attack. The patient is in danger if he makes any sudden flexion movement—for example, at tennis.

Nuclear displacement. Lumbago can also come on in another way. The patient, say, digs in the garden all one afternoon. That evening his back feels vaguely stiff. Next morning he finds himself quite unable to get out of bed, because of severe lumbar pain on the slightest movement. He stays in bed some days and improves; he is up and about after a week and pain-free in another week. The protrusion had increased in size during the night (in other words, what started to ooze out in the afternoon had reached its maximum bulk only by the next morning). This account indicates the soft nuclear type of disc-lesion. Cartilage clicks out suddenly: pulpy protrusions enlarge slowly.

Although the manner of onset indicates whether the consistency of the disc protrusion is hard or soft, the signs found upon examination are identical in either case: a badly blocked joint and compression of the dura mater. Some lumbar movements are very restricted, others not; a cough hurts; and bending the head forwards and straight-leg raising are painful. After some days or weeks of recumbency, the nucleus has oozed back into place again, as the result of the cessation of compression of the disc by the body weight.

After recovery, the patient finds that he can bend up and down quickly—for example, at tennis—without harm; but that if he maintains a flexed posture for a long time, for example, sits with the back unsupported, he is apt to develop backache some hours later, or starting even next day. Yet he can do anything in which the flexed position is held merely momentarily—the opposite of the situation with a cartilaginous disc lesion.

Sciatica

It must be remembered that, when the fourth or fifth lumbar disc protrudes to one side, the pain spreads more or less along the course of the sciatic nerve—that is, along the back of the thigh, the calf, often to the foot. When the third disc protrudes against the third nerve root, the pain is felt instead along the front of the thigh and the front of the leg to just above the ankle. No popular name exists for this condition, since "sciatica" is appropriate only when either of the lower lumbar discs is responsible for pain radiating down the back of the limb (see Figure 1:7).

Root pain can appear in two different ways: primary and secondary.

Primary sciatica. The patient is usually young: eighteen to thirty. He finds that sitting a while makes the buttock and the back of one thigh hurt. A month later, the calf hurts too, still only on sitting. For the next few months he has an ache from buttock to ankle all the time he is upright. The ache becomes worse on sitting, but is absent in bed. A cough hurts the thigh. No pins and needles or numbness are to be expected. Untreated, the condition recovers spontaneously in nine to twelve months. The pain is never severe; the patient is never bedridden nor indeed disabled from any but heavy work.

The signs are merely inability to bend forwards because of pain felt down the lower limb. Straight-leg raising is restricted to about 45 degrees on the bad side, but is of full range on the good side; this becomes evident at the end of the second month or so. The tests for conduction along the compressed nerve root disclose no deficit.

Secondary sciatica. This is apt to affect somewhat older individuals: those aged twenty-five to sixty. The patient has usually suffered several attacks of lumbago in the past. However, this time, just as the pain was leaving the back, he developed instead severe pain down the whole limb. This sequence implies that, the protrusion, at first central and therefore impinging upon the dura mater, has now shifted to one side. The dural tube is thus relieved of pressure at the same moment as the nerve-root becomes pinched. Considerable impact leads to pins and needles or numbness in the toes. (If the third nerve is badly pinched, the numb area is down the front of the leg from knee to ankle.) The pain may be very severe and sometimes is so bad as to compel rest in bed with morphia for the first few days.

After some weeks of severe pain, the leg gradually begins to hurt less, and after two weeks to two months the patient is able to start getting up. Complete spontaneous cure may take a year, but the severest cases with numbness and muscle weakness usually recover much faster than those with a more gradual onset, less severe pain and less advanced signs.

The signs relate to: (*a*) the joint, (*b*) the dura mater, (*c*) the sheath of the nerve root, (*d*) conduction along the nerve root.

The patient stands and visible asymmetry is noted. A tilted vertebra indicates a posture designed to make room for a displacement within the joint. In such a case, one or other of the spinal movements usually hurts to one side of the back. Bending forwards is nearly always restricted by the intensification of the pain in the lower limb.

The patient is then asked to lie on his back. The nerve roots at and below the fourth level are now stretched by raising the leg with the knee straight; this tests the mobility of the sciatic nerve roots (see Figure 2:3). In the case of the third nerve root, stretching involves the patient's lying prone and having his knee bent till his heel approaches his buttock (see Figure 2:4). Restriction of either of these movements indicates impaired mobility—that is, impact against the root. When the nerve has been stretched as far as it will go, the patient is asked to bend his head forwards, thereby stretching the dura mater from above, often with consequent increase of the pain in the limb. Finally, conduction is assessed by testing the strength of the relevant muscles, the sensitivity

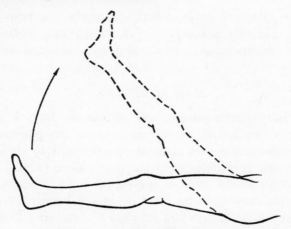

FIGURE 2:3 STRAIGHT-LEG RAISING

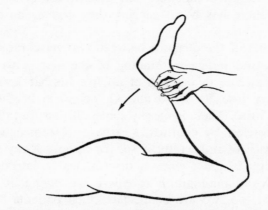

FIGURE 2:4 STRETCHING THE THIRD ROOT

of the skin and the state of the tendon reflexes.

The larger the displacement, the more will it impair the capacity of the nerve root to transmit impulses. Hence, an accurate estimate of the size of the protrusion is not difficult. If the leg cannot be raised far, but conduction is normal, it is fairly small. A larger protrusion interferes both with stretching the root and with conduction. An enormous protrusion may press so hard on the nerve root as to numb it; if so, after a few days of really severe symptoms, the pain ceases; straight-leg raising becomes of full range; but great muscle weakness and insensitivity of the skin become manifest.

X-ray photographs

The ordinary X-ray photograph affords no positive help in assessing a disc-lesion, as it cannot show the position of a fragment of cartilage—a structure transparent to these rays. Its proper use is in differential diagnosis. Since painful *muscle* disease in the spinal areas is almost unknown, a lesion found to affect the moving parts must lie in the bone or the joint. This is just what X-rays can be used to ascertain; they show up bony disease clearly. These rays, therefore, possess an important negative function, but once a confident diagnosis of disc trouble has been reached, they convey no added information.

Narrowing of the distance between two vertebrae is visible, of course, and indicates thinning of the disc. This is sometimes so extreme in old age at all five lumbar levels that a patient may lose 50 or 60 mm (2 inches) in height, but no symptoms arise. There is merely some stiffness that the subject scarcely notices. By contrast, a large displacement may issue from a space of full width; if so, the normal X-ray finding is most deceptive. Even when a disc is clearly causing trouble and the X-ray photograph reveals a narrowing, it does not follow that the two are connected. Such patients have been operated on and have been found to show no evidence of protrusion at the level of the thinned joint-space, but of protrusion from an adjacent disc, radiographically normal. An American surgeon, investigating lumbar disc-lesions by injecting radio-opaque fluid into each spinal joint, found almost twice as many protrusions originating from those with a normal, as opposed to a narrowed, space.

Degeneration of the disc from old age or, precociously, after injury leads not only to thinning but to its bulging out in a circular fashion all round the joint. This pulls on the ligaments that join one vertebral body to the next, and lifts up the membrane lying between the ligament and the edge of the bone. In consequence, since bone grows to meet its limiting membrane, a bony spike called an osteophyte forms. As has already been pointed out, this is a perfectly harmless phenomenon; indeed, it is an advantage, since the weakened disc is now cupped in hard bone rather than soft ligament. Dockers who have carried weights on their backs every day for many years develop large osteophytes and thus keep out of lumbar trouble. The same applies to the joints of the neck in the Portuguese fishwives who carry heavy baskets on their heads (up to 30 kg; 66 lb) every day. Though it is true that at the joints of the limbs these outcrops of bone often signify pain arising from the joint, this does not apply to the spine, otherwise all elderly people would suffer increasing discomfort in the neck and lower back. It is thus very fortunate that the joints of the spine are among those where osteophytes cause no discomfort. The only exception is at the uppermost two, those between skull and first and second vertebrae, which are the only ones that do not contain a disc. Here they may cause early morning headache, easily relieved by manipulation.

What matters in disc-work is whether the fragment is *in* or *out of* place. A displacement in a normal or an abnormal joint hurts, whereas there are no symptoms when there is no displacement, even if the joint is narrowed and osteophytic. This is the very event that the X-rays cannot disclose, and a photograph taken before, during and after an attack of lumbago or sciatica, or of "brachial neuritis" reveals no change. (The same applies to the footballer's knee when the cartilage is torn and displaced; the X-ray photograph merely shows the bones to be normal.)

A displaced disc can be demonstrated on X-ray by a more elaborate technique—myelography—whereby oil is injected into the spinal fluid. By tilting the recumbent patient alternately head up and feet up, the oil is made to flow up and down inside the dural tube. If this investigation reveals a fill-

ing defect, a block is clearly present. However, a disc pro-
truding well to one side may pinch the nerve, yet lie too far
away from the centre to indent the tube; thus, it will not
show up. Hence, even this investigation, when it proves negative, is by no means infallible and it cannot be inferred from
normal myelographic appearances that no disc protrusion is
present. Moreover, just out of interest, a radiologist in the
USA, who was carrying out oil-contrast X-rays for suspected
brain-tumour, let the oil run down to the lumbar area to see
what showed. In 30 per cent of these patients, none of whom
had had back trouble, a defect was visible. Positive findings,
therefore, are not always conclusive either. This brings us
back to the original conclusion: that in disc trouble the main
reliance throughout is on clinical criteria obtained by examining the patient himself.

3

Traditional Treatment

It is remarkable what little effect the discovery of disc-lesions has had on the ordinary treatment of pain in the neck, chest or back, or of "brachial neuritis" and sciatica. In former times, such symptoms were thought of as inflammatory diseases of muscles and nerves ("fibrositis" or "neuritis"). Treatment directed to the muscles followed logically from this erroneous concept. Nowadays, these pains are considered to stem from the joint, but methods of treatment that possess a purely traditional justification are still widely practised.

Cervical disc-lesions

Today, the usual approaches to neck trouble caused by a disc-lesion are: creating disquiet, heat and massage, exercises, traction, a collar.

Creating disquiet
In former days, pains in the neck and shoulder-blade were named "fibrositis." This was an error, but at least not alarmist. It merely led to treatment being given in vain to a secondary phenomenon (the alleged muscle trouble), avoiding the causative disc-displacement. Now that "fibrositis"

has been discredited (Cyriax, 1948), the name that often replaces it is "cervical spondylosis." This misconception is much more difficult to dispel, for the X-ray picture of anyone's neck, if he is middle-aged, is almost certain to show a bony outcrop somewhere, most often at the fifth level, and some erosion of disc substance as well. Hence the radiographic appearances are regarded as confirming the presence of a disease that can only get inexorably worse, and the patient gloomily regards the matter as settled beyond all doubt. It is easy to picture the patient's delight, and his doctor's surprise, when a few treatments by a lay manipulator shift the displaced fragment of disc and abolish the symptoms. A bony spike and an eroded disc are indeed irreversible phenomena, but any patient whose pain comes and goes, or is felt to one side of the neck only, can be sure that these changes are unconnected with his pain. They were present months ago when he had no symptoms, and will still be there months after his symptoms have ceased. Only in the very advanced case, a stage that only a few elderly patients ever reach, is spondylosis really the cause of the trouble.

An alternative label, which also frightens the patient, is "spinal arthritis." It suggests to many people future painful crippledom. Again, it has no more connection with bouts of pain than has the alternative "cervical spondylosis." Another potentially upsetting statement is that "disc degeneration" has set in. Of course it may have set in; almost every healthy middle-aged person has one or more degenerate discs visible on the X-ray photograph. But degeneration without displacement causes no symptoms and is compatible with reaching a ripe old age in comfort.

We have moved from one misnomer to another. "Fibrositis" led to misdirected treatment. The other names lead to mistaken ideas of incurability. Only when acceptance becomes widespread that the symptoms nearly always arise from a displaced fragment of disc can rational treatment come to the fore, and the way lay manipulators achieve their successes be understood. Whether the joint looks normal on the X-ray plate or not, an effort should be made in all suitable cases to get the loose fragment back into place.

Heat and massage

Both are harmless measures, left over from the days when what was in fact disc trouble was thought to result from muscular inflammation. Both afford transient palliation; neither does the slightest lasting good, since the tender spot in the muscle is merely the site of referred pain, not the site of the lesion.

Exercises

By contrast, these are harmful. When the neck is passively rotated during strong traction, the manipulative attempt is carried out while the joint surfaces are held apart; in consequence, *centripetal* force is exerted on the disc. When the patient stands up and carries out what appears to him the same movement, he is turning his head while the joints of the neck bear weight; in other words, *centrifugal* force is acting on the disc. The result of these two separate ways of rotating the neck are, therefore, the opposite of each other. After manipulation has succeeded, *no* exercises should be ordered "to maintain range:" they are likely to have the opposite effect.

The only way to render neck exercises beneficial is to carry them out in a bath, while the head is floating in water.

Traction

This is a reasonable treatment, but so much less effective than manipulation during traction that it need seldom be considered. But it is logically defensible, not of course for "cervical spondylosis," which it cannot reverse, but in the hope of eventually shifting a displacement.

Traction can be given in different ways. The patient may sit with a collar under his chin attached to a spreader and a rope, which passes over a pulley. When the bight is hauled down, his head is lifted and the body weight acts as counter-poise. A similar apparatus can be used with the patient lying on a sloped couch. The rope from the spreader passes almost horizontally to a pulley beyond which hangs the weight. Another alternative is provided by a machine with curved plates, which bear on both shoulders, and two rods, which rise vertically from the plates past each ear. A crossbar moves in a groove along each rod and is attached to the collar. The cross-bar is now pumped upwards, stretching the neck (see Plate 4). Traction by itself is useful only occasionally, but is the best that can be done when manipulation during traction is unavailable.

A collar

This keeps the neck still. Since it stops the patient moving his head, it is often prescribed when the neck movements hurt, and has the effect of preventing the performance of the painful movement. But the real treatment in such a case is to restore painless movement by manipulation; only in the infrequent cases where this endeavour fails completely need a collar be considered at all. Many patients with inter-mittent disc displacement suffer bouts of pain that recover spontaneously. Wearing a collar neither hastens nor delays this relief; some try a collar for a few days; most prefer not to.

There are two logical uses for a collar. The first is to main-tain in place an unstable loose fragment. After painless move-ment has been restored by manipulation, the collar is put on at once. The second is in cases of adherence of the dura mater to the vertebrae. In this uncommon event, bending the neck forward is harmful and the collar is worn indefinitely.

Thoracic disc-lesions

Little traditional treatment exists for pain felt in the chest caused by disc trouble. If it was felt at the back of the chest, it used to be thought of as "fibrositis" and treated by massage to the muscles, and by injections into such tender areas of the unaffected muscles as chanced to be found. Alternatively, if the patient happened to have an asymmetrical or a rounded backbone, he was made to perform postural exercises. If the pain radiated to the front of the chest, it was more likely to be termed "intercostal neuritis" or "pleurodynia" and to be regarded as an obscure and more or less intractable condition which sometimes ceased by itself in the end. Hence, patience and bed-rest were often enjoined.

Lumbar disc-lesions

The normal conservative measures employed for a lumbar disc-displacement consist of: reassurance, rest in bed, heat and massage, exercises, a plaster jacket, a corset. If all these fail and the symptoms warrant, operation is sometimes contemplated.

Reassurance

It is very odd that the X-ray appearances in the neck often serve to increase disquiet, whereas in the lower back they are used to allay concern. Reassurance involves taking an X-ray photograph and informing the patient that no bone disease is present. This policy provides a very simple way of dealing with other people's pain. Admittedly, it does help those who fear that their discomfort denotes cancer, and, for a while, puts neurotics' minds at rest, too. Paradoxically enough, the longer their symptoms last, the more convinced neurotic sufferers become that some serious disease must be responsible. The reverse is actually the case; no important disorder can go on for years without declaring itself.

Reassurance is no help to the individual who wants to lose the pain in his back or leg, not because of anxiety about serious disease, but from a desire to avoid unpleasant symptoms and to return to doing the ordinary things he used to do.

Rest in bed

This has been the standard measure since time immemorial. A doctor in the USA (Browse, 1965) states: "The bed is often the sign of our therapeutic inadequacy, rather than a therapeutic measure deserving praise. The bed is the non-specific treatment of our time, the great placebo." The prescription of recumbency is based on the attitude criticised in Chapter 7, namely, that the patient will get well in the end and that time does not matter. In lumbago, rest is eventually effective in almost every case; it is also, nearly always, a great waste of time. In sciatica, lying down usually eases the pain, perhaps fully, and in the most acute stage may be unavoidable. But, as will be mentioned, the intrasacral injection affords relief much more rapidly. Patients may go on in pain for months or even years in spite of several periods of prolonged rest in bed. Recumbency is certainly no help if the leg has been hurting for longer than a few weeks.

In lumbago it has been alleged that letting the displaced fragment of disc slide slowly back into place during recumbency results in its lying in a more satisfactory situation than that achieved quickly by manipulation. This is not so; in fact, my figures for the incidence of recurrence after manipulation are exactly the same as those of the advocates of rest in bed. The other idea behind rest in bed is to allow the disc to heal, but, as has been explained, this is not possible because two cartilaginous surfaces—being bloodless—can never unite.

Lumbago. As soon as the joint is relieved of the body weight, the centrifugal force acting on it diminishes greatly. The protrusion recedes slightly there and then, and pain is eased at once. The patient is usually kept lying down until the protrusion is all but back in place. This fact is signalled by straight-leg raising returning to full range and coughing becoming painless. The patient is then allowed up for a short while, and later for longer periods, provided that remaining upright does not tend to bring the pain back again. After one to four weeks, nearly all patients have fully recovered.

A patient with lumbago must understand that he can stand and lie, but must not sit. Hence, when he first gets tentatively up, he must walk or remain standing. Sitting can be safely resumed only when he is quite well.

Whether the patient lies flat in bed or on his side, he must keep his back arched throughout. He must on no account sit up, for the body weight now compresses the joint, causing the lumbar spine to assume the convex position that encourages further protrusion. If he lies on his back, a rolled-up towel or a hot-water bottle should support the concavity of his lumbar spine. A good position, if he can keep it up, is lying prone, since this automatically hollows the back. Posture in bed is elaborated in Chapter 6.

That recumbency will allow the loose fragment to return to its proper position is much less certain after the age of sixty; for by then bony outcrops and ligamentous contracture often combine to prevent the bones moving apart when the compression due to body weight ceases. Hence, the older the patient is, the more restricted his lumbar movements are, and the more degenerative changes and bony outcrops the X-ray photograph shows, the more he needs manipulation rather than recumbency for his lumbago. This is the exact opposite of what would be expected and, indeed, of what is widely believed.

Disadvantages of rest in bed. In the case of lumbago these are manifold, and adversely affect the patient, the community and the doctor.

First, the patient has to suffer pain, disablement and loss of earnings for longer than is necessary; moreover, a member of his family may have to stay at home, perhaps off work too, to look after him. Recumbency thus condemns a man to pain lasting days or weeks, during which he has to be nursed. While in bed, though in pain, he is not ill in himself. He therefore maintains his clarity of thought and time passes slowly for him. He lies there, contemplating his sorry plight, and becoming increasingly impatient at the apparent absence of effective treatment. The proper attitude is exasperation, but in patients less emotionally stable, as their minds range, thoughts of incurability may begin to take root; now anxiety, sometimes leading to neurosis, is engendered. If the attack started at work, the idea of industrial compensation begins to loom (see Chapter 8). None of this chain of events would have started if prompt and effective treatment had led to a swift recovery and return to work.

Second, there is the financial loss to the community, which pays the patient sickness benefit, and to the sufferer's employer who loses production and may also continue to pay wages or salary.

Third, there is the loss to the doctor in both esteem and time. If the patient is now treated by a lay manipulator who puts him right, the medical profession is made to look foolish. If the doctor pays him two visits the first week, and one weekly for three weeks after that—five minutes driving there, ten minutes with him, five minutes to the next house on his round—this amounts to a hundred minutes. Examination followed by manipulation cannot take more than half that time. Hence, the very recumbency that appears to save the doctor trouble, in the end wastes his time, too.

Sciatica. When the pain from a disc-lesion is felt in the leg, not the back, the position is rather different. In lumbago, there is only one way in which the patient can get well: by the loose fragment returning to its proper position. In sciatica, there are two possibilities. The loose fragment may go back into place in a manner analogous to the mechanism in lumbago. However, the displacement may become so large that it exceeds the size of the joint aperture; now it can no longer retrace its course. This event means that the patient will be in pain for months, and that he will often find his pain is least when lying down. Since recovery takes place by eventual shrinkage of the protrusion, he has to pass the time pending the completion of this process as best he can. The displacement is maximal, so it will not become larger whatever the patient does after the first few weeks; he lies in bed purely for the relief of pain. He can therefore get up as soon as he likes, whether straight-leg raising is restricted or not, ignoring any numbness or weakness that may have appeared. He will get well at the same rate whatever he does, short of severely straining his back; the whole endeavour is to secure the greatest degree of comfort in the meanwhile. Provided he avoids those postures or activities that increase the pain in the leg, he can do what he likes.

Heat and massage

Heat is comforting. It is therefore suited to alleviating unavoidable pain. It has no place in dealing with a relievable lesion, which should instead be relieved. On a desert island, the best that could be done for a patient with appendicitis might be heat to the abdomen, but this is not the normal approach. The same applies to disc trouble. It may feel nice to have the skin and muscles that overlie a disc displacement warmed up, but the relief is purely subjective and ephemeral.

Radiant heat reaches to a depth of less than 10 mm. Shortwave diathermy and microwaves reach further within the body, and could in theory warm the disc itself. If so, the patient would have a warm displacement which, when the electrodes were removed, would go cold again. Since the dura mater or the nerve root is bruised from the impact of disc material, deep heat has the disadvantage of increasing local oedema—the very opposite of what is wanted.

The idea underlying heat is left over from the days of "fibrositis," when the muscles were really thought to be inflamed. Heat increases circulation and is thus useful in septic conditions, but there are no germs to kill off in disc trouble.

Massage to the muscles has been practised for centuries and may afford some temporary comfort. But there is nothing the matter with the muscles and treatment of them is directed to the wrong tissue. It has been argued that massage serves to relieve painful spasm of the muscles. This is also a faulty idea. The pain, though it is felt in the muscles, does not originate from them. Moreover, the muscles of the back are not in spasm. When they contract strongly they pull the trunk fully backwards, whereas in lumbago the patient holds himself bent slightly forwards. Hence there is no painful spasm to abolish.

Exercises

Heat is harmless enough, but exercises do damage. If they are carried out while the protrusion is in being, this is ground against adjacent tissues and pain is increased. If they are performed when the loose fragment is fully in place, they move the joint about, maintaining the very mobility that predisposes to relapse. The only beneficial exercise is to use the muscles to keep the joint still. A constant postural tone must be inculcated so that the affected joint is kept motionless in the good position—that is, with the back held hollow.

Exercises are often prescribed on the principle that the stronger the muscles, the more stable the joint. This applies

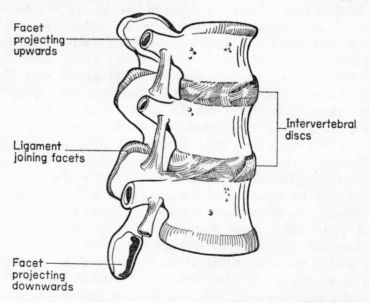

Facet projecting upwards

Intervertebral discs

Ligament joining facets

Facet projecting downwards

FIGURE 3:1 THE FACET JOINTS, LIGAMENTS AND DISCS

to some joints, but not to those of the spine; for here it is not the joint that is unstable, but the loose fragment within it. In fact, the stability of the lumbar joints depends on the ligaments and the apposition of the lateral facets, not the muscles (see Figure 3: 1).

A plaster cast

This may be applied as an emergency measure and is occasionally justified if a patient must be up and about during the first few days of acute lumbago. But, even then, the real answer is to get the loose fragment back into place again by manipulation.

For the prevention of recurrence, a plaster cast is of no help, for it cannot be worn indefinitely. After a few months it must be removed, leaving the loose fragment as loose as it was before. It has the further disadvantage that it cannot be made to fit really well, because the patient could not then breathe after a meal. As a result, it has to be applied too loose. A plastic jacket is adjustable, hygienic and weighs a tenth of a plaster cast; moreover, it can be worn for as long as is necessary (see Plate 5). It should replace the plaster cast entirely.

A corset

Corsets have a bad name with patients, because they are often prescribed wrongly. A corset cannot *put* anything back into place, but it can *keep* something in place. It is therefore required when the loose fragment has been put back into position, or has gone back spontaneously, and has to be kept there. Considerable instability or the wish to continue at heavy work despite a disc-lesion calls for such support.

The object of the corset is twofold – to maintain the lumbar hollow and, as far as possible, to prevent the joint moving. The steel strips must therefore be accurately moulded to fit the convexity of the buttocks and the lumbar concavity. In front, the upper edge of the corset must project far enough above the edge of the lower ribs to catch there if the wearer bends forwards. The two strips must be of metal stout enough to retain their shape when the patient strains against them, moving the wrong way.

No space may intervene between the corset and the patient's back. To make sure that this is so, the fitter kneels behind the standing patient. Her fingers encircle each flank, and each thumb is applied to the steel strip at its point of greatest concavity. She then tries to press both strips against the patient's trunk. If the fit is perfect, she cannot because there is no gap. If they give and bend further to reach his body, they are not properly curved and must be altered. Straight strips follow the curve of the buttocks and bend the unhappy patient's back forwards instead of keeping it hollow, making him worse.

4

Spinal Manipulation

The ideal conservative treatment for all displacements is to return them to their proper position again. This is a doctor's first thought when dealing with a bony dislocation, most fractures or the cartilage in the knee. This intention also governs the choice of treatment in, say, an abdominal hernia or a baby the wrong way up in the womb. Hence, the logical immediate approach to a displaced fragment of disc is, clearly, manipulative reduction. Indeed I know of only one reason for manipulating a spinal joint (except the two uppermost joints of the neck): the restoration to its proper position of a displaced fragment of disc. Once this diagnosis has been reached at a cervical, thoracic or lumbar level, the question of immediate conservative treatment, that is, manipulative replacement, arises. The present logical attitude exhibited towards displacements at the joints of the limbs should now be extended to the spinal joints, and would have the effect of avoiding much prolonged disablement.

Examination

The X-ray picture
In differential diagnosis between disease of bone and other disorders, the X-ray picture has an important part to play.

61

But, once a diagnosis of displacement of part of the disc has been reached, the radiograph offers no further assistance. A diminished joint space may be seen, but attrition of the disc causes no symptoms, nor can it be inferred that any displacement present lies at the particular joint where disc degeneration has occurred. Osteophytes may be visible, but again cause no symptoms; for, as has been established, they cup the disc in bone and tend to diminish the likelihood of displacement occurring. Spondylolisthesis may be revealed. This deformity often leads to a disc-lesion within the unstable joint; in these cases the disc is treated on standard lines, ignoring the spondylolisthesis. By contrast, large displacements of part of the disc often occur, particularly in the young, in radiographically normal joints.

Operation may show that the protrusion lies not at the joint found narrowed, osteophytic or spondylolisthetic, but at the joint just above or below, which appears normal in the X-ray. Excessive reliance on X-ray appearances has another danger. Since most middle-aged people have lumbar osteophytes, it is important not to regard psychoneurotic backache in elderly patients as organically determined because osteophytes are seen, and conversely not to regard young people's organic lesions as trivial merely because radiography reveals nothing.

Clinical examination

This is carried out with attention to six criteria. They determine whether the pain is caused by a displaced fragment of disc or some other disease and what type of lesion is present. They also help in the assessment of what sort of patient the sufferer is: stoical, normal or apt to exaggerate his symptoms.

1   *Inspection.* The way the joint is held
2   *Joint signs.* Pain on some active and passive movements, and not on others, in the partial pattern

3   *Muscle signs.* Pain evoked by movement attempted against such resistance that the joint is held motionless

4   *Dural signs.* Pain when the dura mater or the sleeve of the nerve root is stretched from above or from below

5   *Cord signs.* Conduction along the spinal cord

6   *Root signs.* Condition along a nerve root

Manipulation is indicated if this examination discloses a small cartilaginous displacement at a cervical, thoracic or lumbar joint. The reasons for not manipulating are: that the protrusion is dangerously or awkwardly placed, that it is too large to go back, that it is too long-standing or that it consists of nuclear material and is therefore too soft.

The list of minimum diagnostic procedures makes it clear, I hope, that reading this book is no substitute for a full medical consultation. Moreover, no individual can expect a full clinical examination of this sort from a lay manipulator, who has not followed the medical course that enables him to understand the method and the significance of each finding. Even, therefore, if a patient is determined to visit a lay manipulator, he is earnestly advised to go to his doctor first to ensure that it is safe and reasonable to do so.

Manipulation

If examination reveals a suitable disc displacement, manipulation follows at once. At the joints of the neck and the back of the chest, strong traction is applied before final overpressure is given, i.e. manipulation *during* traction. The lumbar joints are so strong that manual traction is too weak to have any effect, and the situation is also different in another way. Displacements at the neck and thorax nearly always consist of cartilage, and are therefore of the sort that can be clicked into position. However, about a third of all displacements causing low backache consist of nuclear material. This is soft and oozes; it can be sucked back into place but not clicked. Hence, at the lumbar spine, there exist two alternative treatments: manipulation *or* traction, depending on the consistency of the protrusion.

Manipulation, especially of the spinal joints, must not be thought of as a huge uncontrolled wrench; it is a sharp movement of tiny amplitude carried out after the position for this manoeuvre has been reached. For example, a normal neck possesses 90 degrees of active rotary movement. Hence, the operator stretches the neck and turns it through 89 degrees. He then begins to feel the tissue resistance that heralds the end of range. At this moment, his hand is ready to move the joint through another two degrees; one degree to reach the normal limit, the final degree to exert over-pressure. At the instant of this final little thrust, his hand serves not only to move the joint but also to gauge what the end of the movement feels like. This sensation tells him whether to press harder or not, and whether a second manipulation in the same direction is likely to help further.

The preliminary movement to be performed is not the one towards the direction of limitation. The pattern of which movements are painful and which not, and whether the joint is held in the neutral position or with deviation sideways, often helps to indicate what sort of manoeuvre should be adopted initially. If nothing very clear emerges, the first technique is chosen on a basis of three criteria: the likeliest to succeed, the least uncomfortable, the most informative. The experienced manipulator distinguishes different sorts of sensations as the movement reaches the extreme of range and his hand is ready instantly to increase or relax the strength behind the movement, depending on the feel of the joint.

The patient is then re-examined. He reports any change in his pain, not only in that constantly present but in that provoked by each spinal movement. The operator notes any change in range of the movements found to be restricted before treatment was begun. Working on a basis of trial, end-feel and effect, the manipulator continues his sequence of manoeuvres, repeating or abandoning a particular technique on a basis of result and end-feel. He therefore assesses the joint afresh after each manoeuvre. This repeated examination gives clear indications on whether to go on or stop, to try harder or more gently, and what kind of technique to employ.

The manipulations I have devised are based on the fact that normal joints move freely, but the blocked joint does not. Hence, the first part of the manoeuvre is to move all the normal joints as far as they will go. When the operator feels that they have reached the limit of their range, he applies his over-pressure. This now falls on the blocked joint, and the displaced fragment tends to shift out of the way— that is, back into position—thus allowing this joint to move fully, too.

Manipulation must not be thought of as painful. Minor discomfort is caused, it is true, but this does not amount to anything that could be described as pain by normally sensitive patients. The manipulation does not consist of forcing the joint the way it will not go, as many people believe. This applies only in the case of joints that have become stiff from adhesions—for example, minor scarring round a ligament limiting its mobility after a severe sprain, or major adhesions after prolonged immobilisation in plaster while a fracture unites. Then the joint does have to be forced in the restricted direction to rupture the bands limiting that movement.

Quite different considerations apply when a displacement has to be coaxed back into position within a spinal joint. The methods then to be employed are no longer so direct or so simple. The approach has to be more subtle. The manoeuvres are now chosen, one by one, on a basis of what has been found in the past to be most likely to succeed in similar cases. For a patient unable to bend forwards because of acute lumbago, no worse treatment could be thought of

E

than an attempt to force this movement, especially under anaesthesia. Indeed, this is the quickest way to provoke a further increase in the size of the protrusion and is by no means free from risk of lasting aggravation.

Manipulation is effective at once or not at all. Such benefit as is going to be obtained is complete in only a few sessions. During the first treatment, it usually becomes clear whether the endeavour to get the loose fragment back into place will succeed or not. If two sessions afford no relief, the attempt should be abandoned. Most patients require only one or two treatments, but it is always reasonable to continue a few more times as long as further benefit accrues each time. Manipulation ceases at once when the symptoms and signs have ceased. Lay manipulators sometimes continue treatment for months; patients must not lend themselves to this practice (see page 145). Allegedly preventive manipulation is harmful. If the loose piece is in place, further manipulation can only increase joint mobility, with enhanced tendency to recurrence.

Manipulative techniques: set and not-set

There are two types of manipulation: *set* and *not-set*. In the former, anaesthesia is often an advantage and, in any case, is never harmful; in the latter, it deprives the operator of essential information, since the patient is unable to cooperate, thus making nonsense of the whole attempt.

Manipulation : set

Though it is often possible in cases requiring a set manipulation to dispense with it, anaesthesia is often a help, is occasionally essential, and is never a hindrance; for the manipulator carries out a set series of movements without reference to the patient. The manipulator knows what he must do, and does it all the more easily and pleasantly for the patient's unconscious and relaxed state. In, let us say, the removal of the appendix or the reduction of a fracture, the patient can take no active part in furthering the manoeuvre. The same applies to a displace fragment of meniscus at the knee: the manipulation continues until the click signalling reduction is felt. It is then an advantage to both if consciousness is abolished. When adhesions at various joints require rupture, nothing the patient can say or do helps the operator.

Manipulation : not-set

The manipulator does not know what technique will be required in any one case; he merely knows how to set about the work. This state of affairs exists when manipulative reduction is to be attempted at a spinal joint. Though clinical examination can often determine within small limits where a displacement lies, it has no power to establish from which part of the joint it has arisen nor which manoeuvre (if any) will restore it to its bed. Hence, a number of techniques has to be tried, and after each the effect on symptoms and physical signs is assessed on the conscious patient. What to do next—whether to go on or stop—depends on what changes are discerned after each attempt during the session. Anaesthesia must therefore be avoided; for it deprives the manipulator of all knowledge of what he is or is not achieving, and of all finesse. Unless he can examine the conscious patient for warning signs, or at least be told by him of an increase in symptoms, he cannot even tell if he is making the protrusion larger.

What technique should be tried next? This depends on the result of previous manoeuvres on the degree of pain and the range of movement—for example, that of straight-leg raising, or of the joint itself tested on the conscious patient. If subjective or objective improvement results, the same method is repeated. If not, another technique is tried. Is the patient being made worse? If so, manipulation is abandoned before appreciable harm has been done. Should manipulation cease? When examination of the conscious patient reveals that a full and painless range has been restored to the affected joint, there is nothing left to do. If it becomes clear that manipulation is not having any effect, the endeavour is abandoned.

Under anaesthesia, all these vital facts are withheld from the operator.

Anaesthesia in manipulation

Anaesthesia ensures muscular relaxation and freedom from pain. It is called for when any manoeuvre is decided upon that without it would afford unreasonable discomfort; or to abolish such muscle spasm as would militate against success. Anaesthesia is therefore essential for the reduction of most fractures or dislocations, in both of which pain and muscle spasm otherwise render an attempt at reduction impracticable. Orthopaedic surgeons, accustomed as they are to these measures being carried out under anaesthesia, have extended this habit to orthopaedic medicine, not always with the happiest results. The justification for mobilisation of the lumbar spine under anaesthesia rests on a misapprehension of the lesion present. To put a joint through its full range of movement during complete muscular relaxation restores mobility by breaking adhesions. But in backache the pain on, or limitation of, movement is caused not by adhesions but by a block owing to a displacement within the joint, requiring reduction. Admittedly, reduction may occur during mobilisation under anaesthesia, but only by chance not by judgement, and attended, moreover, by difficulties and dangers avoidable as long as the patient remains conscious.

Manipulation under anaesthesia has another disadvantage; it necessitates a night in hospital. Since patients with backache have been estimated to form one-third of orthopaedic surgeons' practice, were they to manipulate under anaesthesia all those requiring this treatment, their wards would be full of such cases to the exclusion of their proper and more important work. The waste of beds, not to say of space in the theatre and anaesthetists' time, would be such that no surgeon would be able to carry on. The overriding needs of severely injured patients have forced a situation upon orthopaedic surgeons whereby they have neither time nor beds to enable them to manipulate the many who need this treatment. They should be able to depute this work to the physiotherapists working on out-patients in their department but, as long as they are not taught these measures as students, the drift to lay manipulators is inevitable.

The displacement fragment of disc that has previously been reduced under anaesthesia is, in my experience, easily reduced on a second occasion without it. In disc-lesions, it is fruitless to resort to anaesthesia when manipulation without it has failed, since it is not the lack of relaxation that was responsible, but the fact that a protrusion irreducible by manipulation is present.

5

Treatment of Individual Spinal Displacements

Spinal displacements are grouped according to level: cervical, thoracic or lumbar.

Cervical disc-lesions

Acute torticollis

Manipulative reduction seldom proves difficult, but has to be carried out differently in patients under and over thirty. For the first two or three days the untreated patient is in severe pain and may be fit only for rest in bed. The fact that spontaneous recovery takes about ten days should not be allowed to condemn the patient to a policy of inactivity, or to its equivalent: heat, massage or a collar. The methods of osteopathy are useless and, indeed, Stoddard, in his *Manual of Osteopathic Practice* (1969), quite rightly warns against the attempt. The St Thomas's manipulative methods are quite different and are successful.

Under thirty. The patient lies down and strong traction is applied to his neck. The head is then first turned several times in the painless direction; and after that bent sideways, again in the painless direction. As a consequence of this treatment, the constant pain ceases and the head can be held symmetrically without pain, but no rotation or side-flexion in the painful direction is yet possible. The patient lies down again and his neck is now rotated as far as it will comfortably go in the painful direction—as yet not far—and is left so for five minutes. After that, it is turned a little further, and so on, until full rotation has been secured. The same is then done for side-flexion. The patient should leave, pain-free, after two hours. Slight recurrence is probable, and he should be seen again next day.

Over thirty. The manoeuvres need no longer be confined to those in the directions that do not hurt. The neck is manipulated first in the painless direction, then in the painful, in the ordinary way.

Unilateral scapular pain

The pain is felt at one side of the neck and in the shoulderblade area. Within this area lies a tender spot which the patient has found for himself and identifies, mistakenly, as the source of his pain. While doctors have attacked this secondary phenomenon in vain by massage, injections, and so on, lay manipulators have paid no attention to the spot but have merely manipulated the neck. The lay manipulators' treatment, although it often stems from a wrong diagnosis, does stop the pain.

Unilateral pain in the arm

When a disc protrusion in the neck compresses a cervical nerve root at any level between the fourth and the seventh, pain in one arm results. This used to be called "brachial neuritis," which directed attention to the arm, whereas the trouble lies at the neck joint.

Muscle weakness. If the pain is accompanied by muscle weakness, manipulation is useless and the patient has to await spontaneous recovery, which takes three to four months from when the pain radiated to the arm, *not* from when the pain began in the shoulder-blade. Meanwhile, strong pain-killers are required.

No muscle weakness. Pain down the arm without muscle weakness indicates a smaller protrusion, and about half of all such displacements can be put back by manipulation if they are seen within the first two months of the onset of pain in the limb. The others have to wait the four months.

Acroparaesthesia

The ache is not severe but is felt in both arms, with pins and needles in both hands. Manipulation of the neck is sometimes effective.

Pins and needles in hands and feet

When this is caused by a central disc protrusion in the neck, manipulation consists of strong manual traction without rotation. It sometimes succeeds. If it does not, a collar may help. A few patients require operation eventually.

Thoracic disc-lesions

These are usually easy to put back, but are also inclined easily to recur, and most patients have to attend again for manipulative treatment, perhaps yearly. As at the neck, manipulation of the spinal joints at the back of the chest is carried out during traction.

The rules for manipulating and not manipulating that apply to the neck and lumbar joints do not apply here, and almost all small protrusions can be put back in one or two sessions, whether the pain is at the back of the chest, the front, or both.

Manipulative technique

The patient lies prone, one assistant grasping the hands, another the feet. They pull hard and the patient consciously relaxes; the bones come apart slightly and room is created for the loose fragment to move.

Various types of pressure are given at the level of the

displacement. A quick small jerk is applied downwards in different ways. Re-examination then follows. If necessary, the operator passes on to rotary manoeuvres.

Lumbar disc-lesions

In my experience, two-thirds of all patients with backache and onet-hird of all those with sciatica are relievable by manipulation. A small displacement, consisting of cartilage, is suited to manipulation, but if it consists of soft nuclear material, traction must be substituted. The lumbar joints are so large and strong that manipulation has been found no more effective during manual traction than without it. If manipulation is attempted during mechanical traction, the strong tension on joints and muscles makes the back so rigid that all movement is prevented and nothing is achieved. It is therefore a question of alternatives—manipulation *or* traction—and the choice rests on the decision whether the protrusion is likely to be hard or soft.

Indications for manipulation
Backache felt centrally or to one side of the spine at a low lumbar level should be treated by manipulation when one, two or three of the four lumbar movements hurt. The patient stands and is asked to bend as far as he can backwards, sideways and forwards. These movements should increase the pain, but at least one movement should make no difference. Pain felt when the patient bends half-way forwards, ceasing when the extreme of flexion has been reached, is an encouraging sign. In patients under sixty, pain elicited by bending sideways *towards* the painful side diminishes the likelihood of success, but after sixty it no longer has this significance.

Lumbago, i.e. pain in the back coming on suddenly and severely, should *always* be treated by manipulation unless the case is hyperacute and the attempt too painful to be borne, in which event the patient requires epidural local anaesthesia (described later in this chapter). Whether straight-leg raising is of full range or is limited makes no difference.

In sciatica, the patients who do best are those who have pain both in the back *and* down the back of the thigh and calf. Age over sixty is a favourable indication.

Indications against manipulation

Naturally, to endeavour to put a fragment of disc into position when it is not displaced is futile. In all backache not caused by disc trouble (and there are many other causes of the complaint, but none is common) manipulation must be avoided. Other reasons are:

1 *Hyperacute lumbago.* Cases are encountered of such severe lumbago that any attempt to move the patient produces agonising twinges. Manipulation would be unbearable. Treatment should be the injection of a local anaesthetic solution into the sacrum betwen the protrusion and the dural tube.

2 *Pressure on the fourth sacral nerve.* This is rare and is signalled by weakness of the bladder, or numbness in the genital area or lower sacrum.

3 *Too large a protrusion.* Muscle weakness, loss of the tendon reflex, or numbness of the skin of the lower limb indicates a protrusion too large to be put back.

4 *Lumbar deviation with sciatica.* Many patients with lumbago have to lean forwards or sideways, holding the joint in such a way as to make room for the displacement. When the pain is purely in the back, this deviated posture by no means bars manipulation, but usually implies that several sessions will be required. However, if the pain is felt only in the limb, and the patient cannot hold himself erect because any attempt to straighten his spine shoots a pain down the leg, all conservative treatment is likely to fail and an operation is usually required. Before deciding, it is worth while trying the epidural injection once.

5 *Sciatica of more than six months' standing.* In patients under sixty years old, the fact that pain in the lower limb, without appreciable backache, has lasted more than six months indicates that it is too late to hope for success by manipulation. These are the very cases that benefit from the epidural injection into the sacrum.

6 *Sciatica without backache.* Sometimes sciatica comes on without premonitory backache, the pain being felt first, perhaps, at the back of the thigh and later spreading to the calf and buttock. Such a protrusion does not respond to manipulation, but traction is effective during the first few months.

7 *Pregnancy.* During the first four months of pregnancy, manipulation can be carried out in the ordinary way. After that, for the next four months, the manipulations involving the patient lying prone cannot be used, but those carried out with the patient lying on her side or her back remain practicable. During the last month, rest in bed is the best treatment.

Manipulative technique

The lumbar joints are too large and strong for manual traction to have an appreciable effect on them. Hence, the traction that is so great a help at the smaller joints of the neck and thorax is no longer applicable. The patient lies prone and the affected joint is identified; a series of sharp pressures towards extension is given. Or he may lie on his side and have his chest rotated one way and his pelvis the other, while the two are stretched apart. Or he may lie on his back and the thigh be used as a lever to give a stronger twist to the pelvis as the final thrust is given. Between each manoeuvre, the patient is re-examined, so that the operator can assess the result of each technique and be guided towards the one that helps that particular patient most. The operator can also tell whether to go on or stop and what to do next. All these methods are illustrated in my book for physiotherapists (*Orthopaedic Medicine*, volume 2).

Traction

There is nothing new about mechanical traction. It was already being used in Turkey in the fifteenth century, and at the Wellcome Museum in London stands a traction couch dating from 1544 (see Plates 7 and 8).

Traction for the replacement of the soft type of disc protrusion was first put forward in Britain (Cyriax, 1950) and our original couch is still in use (see Plate 9). During the last twenty years most hospitals over here have acquired one, and treatment should be given by physiotherapists trained in the different techniques.

The patient may lie on his abdomen or on his back, and for each of these positions there are four different ways of applying the harness, all illustrated in my *Orthopaedic Medicine*, volume 2, each with a slightly different angle of pull on the lumbar joint. In a simple case, any method will do, but when a displacement proves difficult to shift, each of these eight variations may have to be tried, until the effective one is singled out.

The principle is simple: merely to produce a negative pressure within the joint, and to suck back the protrusion. Traction separates the joint surfaces (see Plate 6) and tautens the ligaments, with added centripetal effect. The treatment has to be painless, since the muscles must relax to allow the traction to pull the bones apart. Pain makes the patient tighten his muscles, thus nullifying the effect. If pain is experienced, the traction is either being given the wrong way or an unsuitable lesion has been chosen in error.

The distracting force must be constant. The intention is to stretch out the muscles till fatigue sets in and relaxation allows the vertebrae to come apart. X-ray studies have shown that this begins after two minutes. If intermittent traction is employed, the muscle is stretched and responds by a reflex automatic contraction; hence, the bones do not move apart however often this is done. Many lay manipulators in Britain use intermittent traction with an impressive electric motor. Nevertheless, it is a mistaken policy.

The amount of distraction is the greatest that the patient feels to be pleasantly tolerable. A small woman may need only 40 kg; a really large man may need as much as 90 kg. But the more tension that can be borne without discomfort, the better. This is because the object of the treatment is to draw the nuclear bulge towards the correct position. As soon as the patient gets up, he compresses the joint afresh and squeezes it out in the wrong direction. The distance through which the bulge moves during half an hour of treatment must, therefore, be greater than the distance through which it is squeezed out again during the rest of the day. Hence it is not worth while initiating traction at all unless it can be given daily. In urgent cases, a session morning and late afternoon is warranted, continued until reposition is complete. Most patients begin to improve only after two or three visits; indeed, the patient who is enormously better after one session usually does not do so well in the end as those who improve gradually.

Some patients begin to recover only during the second week; hence, it is reasonable to go on daily for two weeks before giving up. Naturally, if these two weeks have afforded considerable improvement, continuance for a third week, rarely a month, is justified. If one or two sessions of traction increase the symptoms, the method should be abandoned forthwith.

During the traction, the constant ache usually disappears, since the bulge recedes as the bones come apart and the pressure on the dural tube or the nerve root consequently lessens. But traction must not be applied merely till symptoms cease—this might be only a few kilos. This is no criterion. Traction must be increased until the patient feels that it is about as much as he can take without discomfort.

Indications for traction

The reasons for employing traction rather than manipulation are as follows.

1 *Soft protrusion*. A small, hard cartilaginous fragment can

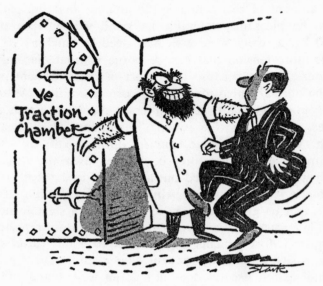

" Given by physiotherapists "

FIGURE 5:1

(*Reproduced by permission of the Arthritis and Rheumatism Council*)

usually be shifted by manipulation. By contrast, manipulation will not affect a soft protrusion. If, then, it is the nucleus that has protruded, it must be sucked back. The situation is analogous to taking a hammer to a nail, but a syringe to syrup.

2 *First and second lumbar disc-lesions.* These are rare, but when they do occur, manipulation usually fails, whereas traction is nearly always effective.

3 *Recurrence after operative removal of the disc.* Renewed protrusion after excision of a protruded disc at laminectomy may result from a further displacement at the same joint, or a new displacement at another level. Manipulation is quite safe, but often fails. By contrast, traction is usually successful.

4 *Manipulation fails.* Cases are encountered where manip-

ulation is confidently begun, but unexpectedly affords no benefit. The reason is usually that a soft protrusion has been mistaken for a hard one. Since the distinction in consistency is difficult to draw, errors occur from time to time. But little is lost, for lack of progress during the first manipulation makes the situation plain. Next day, traction is substituted.

Indications against traction

Traction must never be given in acute lumbago causing sudden sharp accesses of pain on movement. These cases require manipulation or epidural local anaesthesia. Though the patient loses his pain while lying stretched on the couch, unwinding him usually provokes a series of agonising twinges. The distracting force has to be reduced very slowly indeed, and it may take several hours to get the patient off the couch, and even then he remains the worse for his ordeal till next day.

Traction obviously cannot be given to a patient so bent up that he cannot lie flat on the couch.

Traction should not be tried on patients with cartilaginous displacements requiring manipulation.

In old age, the nucleus has ceased to exist. Hence, past the age of sixty, all protrusions consist of cartilage and are thus suited to manipulation, not traction.

In sciatica with signs of muscle weakness, lost reflex or numb skin, the protrusion is larger than the aperture whence it emerged, and neither traction nor manipulation can shift it. Pain in the lower limb, without backache, that has lasted longer than six months, is not at all likely to benefit, nor is a sciatica which bends the patient over so far forwards or sideways that he cannot stand upright (see Plate 1).

Maintenance

Once the damaged part of the disc has returned to its bed, it must be kept there; for what has shifted once will shift again, if the same mechanical conditions are repeated as caused the original displacement.

The patient must henceforth keep his back hollow by: (*a*) maintaining the muscles that straighten the back in a state of slight constant contraction, (*b*) supporting his back properly, especially while sitting, (*c*) having sclerosing injections into the spinal ligaments, (*d*) wearing a belt, (*e*) operative fusion. Alternative approaches in cases of gross instability are: (*a*) injection of chymopapain into the joint, to enable the enzyme to destroy the disc, (*b*) laminectomy, to remove the greater part of the disc.

Sclerosing injections

Ligaments support joints and, if they become slack, the condition can be likened to loose guy-ropes rendering a tent unstable. If they are tightened the tent becomes able to withstand much stronger forces. Improved stability can be secured by sclerosant treatment. The solution used is irritant and contains sugar and phenol. This is injected into the junction between ligament and bone at all the ligaments supporting the damaged joint. Three treatments are given at weekly intervals. The injection induces a chemical inflammation which subsides with consequent local fibrosis. The scar-tissue then contracts. The result of the infiltration is thus the formation of new tough fibrous tissue, with eventual contracture stabilising the joint. Since it is excessive movement towards flexion that needs to be arrested, the ligaments requiring shortening are those lying behind the joint—fortunately the very ones most accessible to a needle. The injection smarts as the fluid is introduced, and the back is sore for the rest of the day. The full effect is not manifest until the scarring is complete; this takes five to eight weeks. Three weeks after the last treatment the patient is asked to walk two miles daily for two weeks, whereupon it is hoped that he can resume normal activities. If any tendency to recurrence is noted, a "booster" injection can be given at whatever intervals prove necessary.

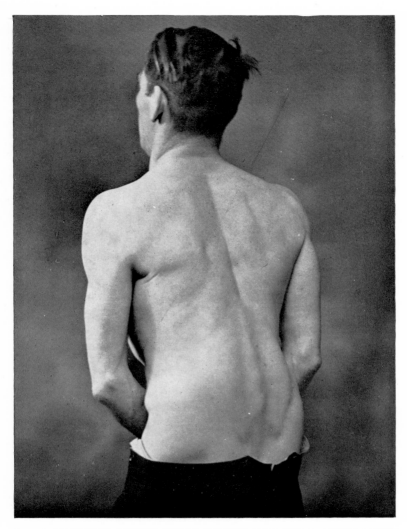

1   A PATIENT FIXED BENT FORWARDS BY A DISPLACED
FRAGMENT OF DISC

This photograph shows him trying to bend backwards. Marked lumbar
deformity caused by posterior protrusion of part of a low lumbar
intervertebral disc with left-sided sciatica. The patient is bending
backwards as far as he can

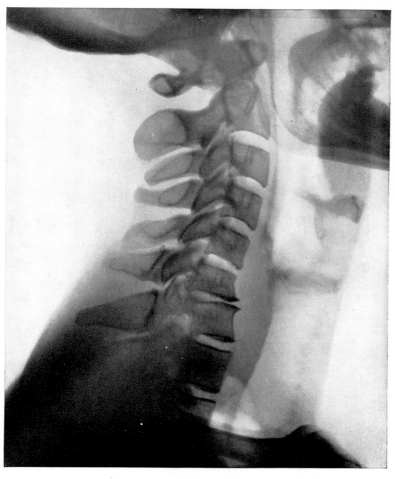

2   CERVICAL DISC LESION

Sixth cervical disc-lesion. Lateral view of cervical spine showing
marked narrowing and tilt at the sixth cervical joint. This contrasts
with the normal spaces above and below

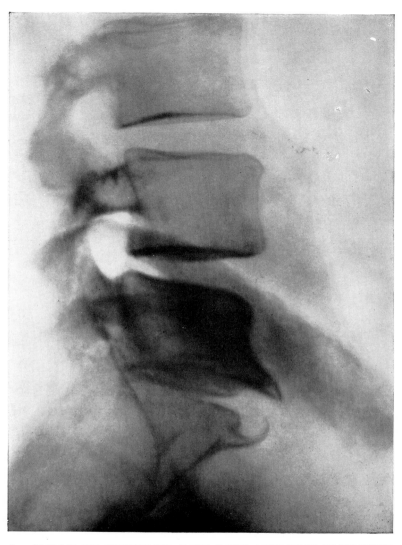

3 X-RAY OF FORWARD DISC DISPLACEMENT ENCLOSED BY BONY SPIKES

Anterior disc protrusion. The fifth lumbar disc has been reduced to rubble and the intervertebral bodies lie in contact. Remaining disc substance has become displaced forwards, where it lies enclosed by the two huge osteophytes that have formed in consequence of the traction exerted by the anterior longitudinal ligament. Since the protrusion does not impinge on a sensitive structure, for many years nothing is felt; finally compression causes the "mushroom phenomenon"

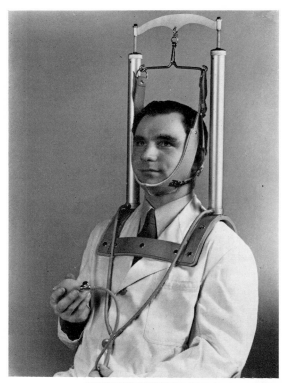

4   ZIMMER NECK
TRACTION APPARATUS

5   PLASTIC
LUMBAR JACKET

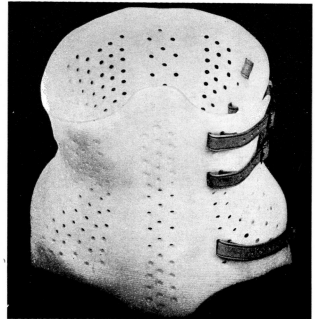

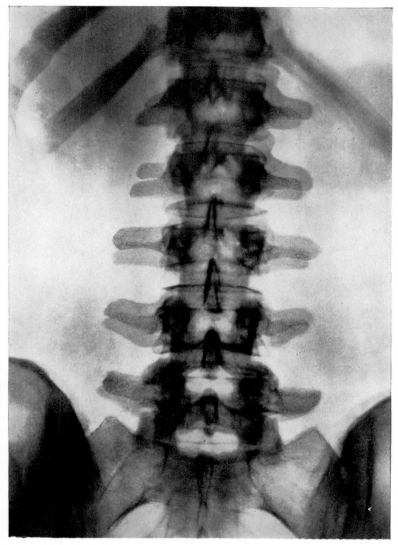

**6   X-RAYS TAKEN BEFORE AND DURING TRACTION ON
LUMBAR SPINE**

Two photographs have been superimposed, corresponding at the
sacrum and iliac crests. The first was taken as the subject lay prone,
the second after ten minutes' traction by 45 kg (100 lb). The amount
of distraction obtained is clearly visible

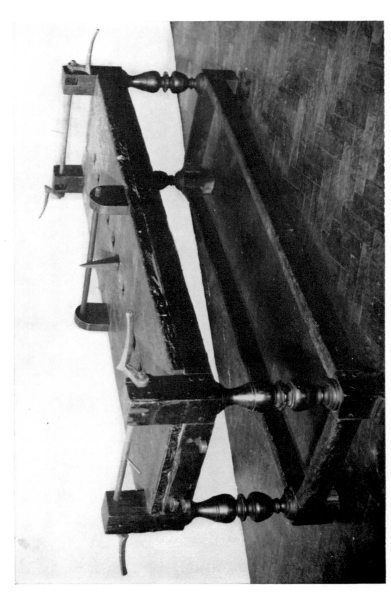

7   EARLY ITALIAN TRACTION COUCH

As used by Hippocrates and illustrated in Guidi's Chirurgia, 1544.
Discovered in 1923 near Urbino, Italy and now in the Wellcome

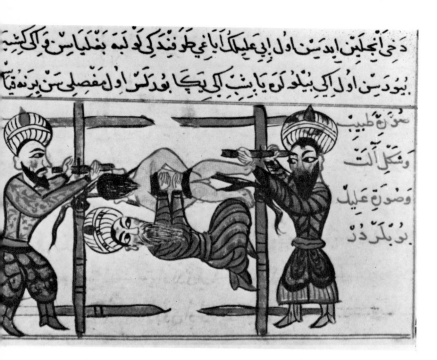

8   MEDIEVAL TURKISH TRACTION

An illustration taken from "Le Premier Manuscrit Chirurgical Turc de Charaf-Ed-Din" (1465)

(*Reproduced by permission of the Bibliothèque Nationale, Paris*)

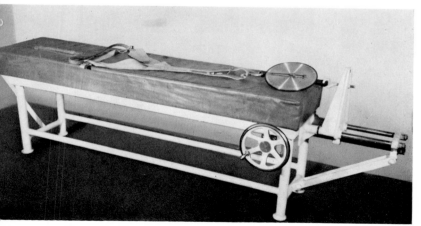

9   MODERN TRACTION COUCH

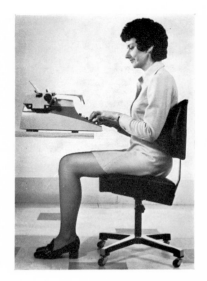
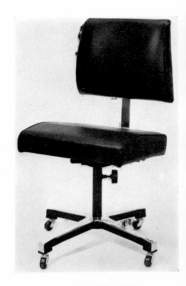

10   A GOOD EXAMPLE OF A TYPISTS CHAIR
(Tan-Sad Chair Company)

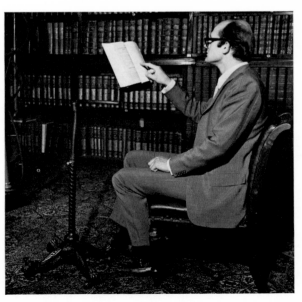

11   A READING STAND AT THE ATHENAEUM
(Reproduced by courtesy of the Athenaeum Club, London)

R. Barbor's figure for lasting relief (followed for up to eight years) is 90 per cent.

Epidural local anaesthesia

This is my third standard method for dealing with lumbar disc-lesions. Whereas spinal manipulation was begun more than 2000 years ago, and traction more than 500, this injection is a comparative newcomer. The technique was invented by Sicard in France in 1901. He pointed out that there was a small aperture at the lower part of the sacral bone which allowed the passage of a needle (see Figure 5:2). Fluid could, therefore, be introduced into the cavity within the sacrum (see Figure 5:3) and thence be made to flow upwards within the spinal canal and downwards along the external aspect of the nerve roots.

The injection consists of inserting a long needle into the sacrum by way of the small aperture lying between the two projections (cornua) at the lowest part of the sacrum. These can be felt and serve as a guide to the channel that the needle must traverse.

Fifty millilitres of a 1:200 solution of procaine are slowly injected. The patient feels first a tension in his lower back; later, if he suffers root pain, the familiar ache in the leg is reproduced. The injection takes about ten minutes and afterwards the patient stays lying down for another fifteen minutes. Some patients feel a little giddy or develop a transitory headache; if so, they lie there for a little longer until the reaction has passed; longer than half an hour is exceptional. They go home in the ordinary way, and come again for reassessment a week later. It is no use their coming earlier; for the effect of the injection over the first two or three days is very variable and the final result is not clear until a week has elapsed.

At the time, no one paid any particular attention to Sicard's discovery, and the injection remained a technical possibility which was put to little practical use. In 1937, while searching

F

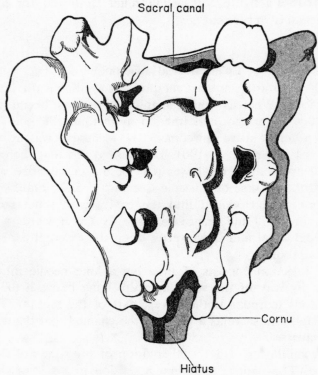

FIGURE 5:2   SACRUM

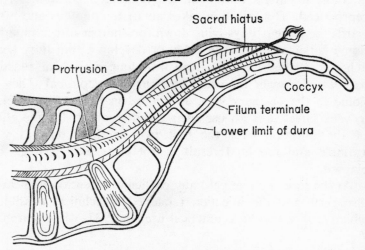

FIGURE 5:3   NEEDLE WITHIN SACRUM (Back of body at the top
of the figure)

for the sources of pain in the back and lower limb, I first began to seek confirmation or disproof of each localisation I had arrived at by injecting a local anaesthetic solution. I then waited to see if the pain would cease for the time being. If I hit the wrong spot, no relief ensued, and I knew that I had to look elsewhere for the origin of the symptom.

It was then that I started to use Sicard's injection into the sacrum, using a dilute solution of procaine. The idea was that the pain would cease if a disc lesion was responsible, but not if any other disorder were present. The argument was that the disc, when it bulged out backwards, squeezed either the dural membrane, causing backache, or the nerve root, causing pain in the limb. Anaesthetisation of only the external aspect of the dura mater and the nerve root would, so it seemed to me, render these two tissues temporarily insensitive and the pain would thus cease for as long as the numbing effect lasted—that is, for one to two hours.

This idea proved correct, and I still use this injection, not only extensively in treatment, but also as a method of confirmation or disproof in difficult cases. The remarkable fact then emerged that many, but by no means all, patients declared, when they were seen a week or two later, that the improvement had been maintained. At first, I was incredulous, regarding the relief as fortuitous. But it did not take long before it became evident that what I had started as an adjunct to diagnosis had transformed itself into a potent method of treatment.

Further experience showed the injection to be useful in the following types of disorder.

1 *Hyperacute lumbago.* The patient lies motionless in bed, entirely unable to move because of agonising twinges at the slightest attempt to do so. He dare not cough or sneeze. In such a case, an attempt at manipulation would be unthinkable; vain, too, since relaxation would be impossible. The only effective treatment is the epidural injection, which causes no appreciable discomfort. Ten minutes after it is finished,

the patient finds to his surprise that he can move perfectly freely without pain. This full relief lasts about an hour and a half, during which period he can move about in bed, but should keep face downwards. Then some discomfort returns, but seldom the severe pain or the twinges. Next day, the patient can usually get up, and any residual ache can be dealt with in the ordinary way by manipulation.

This injection represents the only simple short cut to immediate relief in really severe lumbago (Cyriax, 1945).

2 *Nocturnal or matutinal backache.* Uncommonly, a patient complains of backache only at night or only on waking. By day, whatever he does causes no discomfort. Examination by day reveals nothing; movement at the lumbar joints may prove slightly restricted, but no pain is elicited. The common cause of early morning backache is spondylitis. If this disease has been excluded, clinical examination and X-ray photography reveal no disorder. One epidural injection often stops the ache lastingly.

3 *Incurable backache.* Sometimes disc trouble causes a chronic backache which neither manipulation nor traction abates. A case such as this often benefits from sclerosing injections into the lumbar ligaments but, should these fail, it is sometimes possible so to desensitise the bruised tissues inside the back that the continuous ache ceases. The momentary pain on movement often persists, but is by comparison a minor matter.

4 *Sciatica with impaired conduction.* Once a disc displacement causing pain down the limb has become large enough to cause muscle weakness, numb skin or an absent tendon reflex, both manipulation and traction are bound to fail; for the hernia is larger than the aperture whence it emerged and it cannot go back (see Figure 1:7). The only conservative treatment left, except helplessly to consign the patient to bed for as long as may be, is relief from bruising of the nerve root by means of the intrasacral injection. The fluid

passes between the bulging disc and the nerve root, numbing it. The remarkable fact is that the desensitisation of the nerve root is usually lasting, the pain never returning to anything like its previous level. Another similar injection a week later, with perhaps another a fortnight after that, brings about full recovery from a condition that certainly takes many months, and at times a year, to resolve spontaneously.

It is a widely held belief that evidence of loss of conduction along the pinched nerve root is a good reason for operative removal of the disc. This is not so; I have treated thousands of such cases with the injection, and only a small proportion has ever needed the operation. This is called for only if the pain remains severe and epidural local anaesthesia fails. But so many hospitals contain a surgeon expert in the operation and so few hospitals contain a physician practising this injection that the operation is often regarded as the only effective measure in a case of this type.

5 *Sciatica lasting too long.* Sciatica usually gets well of itself in a year. Cases are encountered now and then of a sciatica that has gone on for much longer—my most chronic successful case had lasted nine years. Unless the nerve root is actually bound down by adhesions (a rarity) the pain ceases after the injection and mobility is restored to the nerve root within a few minutes. Straight-leg raising, which may have been stubbornly restricted for some years, returns to full range at once. Two epidural injections usually bring about lasting recovery.

6 *Bruised nerve root.* Sometimes a disc-lesion may resolve completely to all appearances, or be surgically removed, yet the ache in the limb remains. The lumbar joints move well without causing any discomfort; straight-leg raising is full and painless. In short, examination of the back and of the lower limb reveals nothing. In such cases, the pain appears to be caused by persistent bruising of the nerve root, owing to past compression by a disc protrusion which has now receded. In

these cases, epidural local anaesthesia can be relied upon to desensitise the nerve root at the site of former impact; one injection suffices for lasting relief.

Operation

This is not often required at any lumbar level, since conservative treatment is so often successful. My figure for removal of the disc in sciatica is 3 per cent. At the neck, operation is required more rarely still; at the thoracic levels, hardly ever. Some figures on the frequency of operations for the removal of discs have emerged (Brügger, 1960) from Switzerland. Of 2948 operations, 21 were for cervical, 7 were for thoracic, 20 for first or second lumbar, 135 for third lumbar and 2765 for fourth and fifth lumbar protrusions.

Myelography

This investigation is hardly ever necessary when a lumbar disc is at fault, but is always required before operation on a cervical or a thoracic disc protrusion, in order to establish the exact level. It is not worth carrying out unless, should the findings prove positive, operation is contemplated.

Myelography consists of injecting oil opaque to X-rays into the spinal fluid. Then the patient is placed on a tilting table and the oil watched on the screen as it flows up, then down. Any interference with the flow is then photographed by X-rays. This examination is of great value in distinguishing disc protrusions from other space-occupying lesions within the spinal canal. It is trustworthy in the cervical and thoracic regions, but less so at the lower lumbar levels. The protrusion, in order to indent the dural tube, must project fairly centrally. The two lowest lumbar joints are much wider than those in the neck and at the back of the chest; hence, a protrusion may emerge well to one side, pinching the nerve root severely but not showing up at all on the myelogram. In only about three-quarters of all cases of lumbar disc protrusion does the myelogram display interruption of the flow of oil. Hence, it is usual for surgeons to operate on suitable lumbar cases without this preliminary.

Cervical disc-lesion

When pain down one arm is the main symptom, operation is best avoided altogether.

If signs of pressure on the spinal cord appear, operation may well be the best treatment if the myelogram shows clear indentations—often more than one.

Thoracic disc-lesion

Operation is required in the rare cases of pressure exerted on the spinal cord. The myelogram indicates the level.

Lumbar disc-lesion

Removal of the disc. The indication for laminectomy is intractable pain in a sincere patient. Patients with neurosis often welcome operation, but seldom achieve relief that lasts more than a few months; some allege that they have been worse since the very day that it was carried out. It is immaterial whether examination shows that conduction along the nerve is impaired or not; the indication is genuine severe symptoms that have defied adequate conservative treatment, which includes the induction of epidural local anaesthesia and blocking the sinuvertebral nerve. These injections relieve so many otherwise intractable sciaticas that, in my view, no one should be operated on without their effect being tried at least once. The cases most often qualifying for operation are those with gross lumbar deformity. The lumbar spine deviates considerably, to one side or forwards, and any attempt to straighten the back is prevented by severe pain radiating down the leg.

The other indication for removing the disc is evidence of pressure on the fourth sacral root—that is, numbness in the saddle or genital area, or weakness of the bladder.

It is wise, at laminectomy, if only the fourth or the fifth disc is found to be at fault, to inject chymopapain prophylactically at the undamaged level.

Operative fusion. Arthrodesis, the operation for fusing two vertebrae together by a bridge of bone, used to entail three months in bed followed by another three months up and about in a plaster jacket. Patients were thus very unwilling to undergo surgery, owing to the time factor. Now, only two or three weeks in bed are necessary, for, by means of screws, the joints are held motionless while the graft unites.

Arthrodesis is indicated in: recurrent severe attacks of pain that make the patient's life unmanageable, in forward slipping of one vertebra on the one below (spondylolisthesis), or in compression phenomena.

Two new treatments

Two very promising and novel approaches to disc trouble have recently been made: chemical destruction of the disc and severing the sensory nerves.

Chymopapain

Destruction of the disc by means of an enzyme was put forward by Smith of Chicago in 1963. After extensive animal experiments he evolved a solution and a technique that was 88 per cent successful in a series of cases reported on in 1969. Instead of removing the disc surgically, he injected chymopapain into the disc, which was eaten away in a few hours. The enzyme does not erode adjacent tissues. Smith's work has expanded and there are now over thirty centres where chymopapain is used, with overall complete relief in three-quarters of all cases otherwise requiring surgery. Some 2000 patients have now been treated without a single death attributable to the drug.

The method entails the insertion of a separate needle into each damaged disc during general anaesthesia; it is a skilled operation requiring X-ray control. In the successful cases pain is lost within a day or two and five to seven days in hospital suffice.

For the first time, it has become possible to get rid of a bulging disc without physical removal. Indeed, chymopapain has proved successful in shrivelling discs already subjected in vain to surgery. Complete relief is reported even in a patient who had had laminectomy performed three times without avail.

Smith's original research on chemonucleolysis is clearly proving the most far-reaching advance in disc work for the past twenty years. In the USA his method will be welcomed particularly by the Workmen's Compensation authorities, who have become increasingly concerned at the huge amounts awarded by the courts to injured patients after spinal surgery.

Division of nerves

This is a method devised by Skyrme Rees, an English surgeon working in Australia. He published a booklet describing his work in 1971.

Pairs of nerves, called the posterior rami, emerge from the spine, passing through the same apertures between the vertebrae as house the large nerve roots. One branch doubles back into the spine again, supplying the dura mater, vertebral ligaments and bone with sensory fibres. Another divides into two, one twig serving the adjacent facet joint, the other nearby bone and muscle. Each posterior ramus can be caught just beyond the edge of each vertebra where it lies close to the membrane joining the transverse processes of two adjacent bones (see Figure 5:4).

Here the nerve can be cut by a long thin scalpel, nicking it at the edge of the membrane. Rees has performed this operation a thousand times, all of which, so he claims, were a complete success, with only two exceptions. Extensive trial by other surgeons has yielded 50 to 80% good results.

I have adopted this method, setting about it slightly differently.

My idea has been to inject a local anaesthetic agent into the spot where the nerve emerges to discover where the relevant nerve lies. The patient stands and indicates which movements of his trunk hurt. The injection is given and the movements assessed again. This is continued at different levels until painless movement has been restored—the indication that the solution has numbed the right spot. A sclerosant solution is then injected at that spot. Only if this fails need the nerve actually be divided.

6

Prevention of Disc Trouble

It is worth while taking trouble to avoid, or at least to postpone, the development of a disc-lesion, especially at a lumbar level. People cannot hope to use their lower back the wrong way and get away with it for very long.

The key to the whole problem is the postural maintenance of the normal hollow at the neck and lower back, and keeping the spinal convexity at the back of the chest to a minimum. Set out in this chapter are many activities that imperil the integrity of the intervertebral discs.

Babyhood

Evidence has lately been accumulating that a disorder named spondylolisthesis (which had been regarded as due to an inborn defect in the vertebral arch) is seldom congenital but is acquired during babyhood. Repeated strains fall on the lowest two lumbar vertebrae when a baby is about a year old. Stress fractures form between the two halves of the vertebral arch, but cause no appreciable discomfort. No one realises their presence and union by bone seldom takes place. Fibrous tissue fills the gap—a stretchable structure. After years of tension—some time during adolescence—the defect enlarges. The vertebra becomes longer and grows to project in front of the one below it, out of line. An unstable joint forms between these two vertebrae. In consequence, a precocious disc-lesion results, often during the patient's teens. It is true that not all people with spondylolisthesis have symptoms; nor, if they do, are they always caused by disc-lesions, but this is the case in the vast majority.

Repeated strains cause fatigue fractures in bone in the same way as bending an iron rod first one way and then the other eventually breaks it. The baby not yet able to walk, learns to move about seated, with one leg bent before him, propelling himself with the other leg. At each shove, the buttocks are bumped against the floor while the lumbar spine is held flexed. Alternatively, when a baby first learns to walk after a few steps upright, his legs give way and he lands on his buttocks with the lumbar spine convex. These repeated stresses are now regarded as the main cause of a condition that is found present in about 4 per cent of all patients with backache.

It is therefore important to discourage babies from pushing themselves along seated, and to see to it that they go on crawling till they can walk. The baby who keeps falling seated should be provided with a thick napkin to cushion the fall and give him less far to go. There is a great deal to be said for the various walking machines now on the market, which enable the child to stay upright as he pushes himself along (see Figure 6 : 1).

Posture at school

During the last twenty-five years, the attitude towards young people's posture has gradually had to be reversed. From time immemorial, aesthetic considerations have held sway. Clearly, a hollow back leads to prominence of the abdomen and buttocks, whereas a flat lumbar spine means a graceful carriage and a shapely freedom from bulges in front and behind. But then came the discovery of the disc as the common cause of back troubles and sciatica. This has led to an alternative criterion for the evaluation of posture : no longer

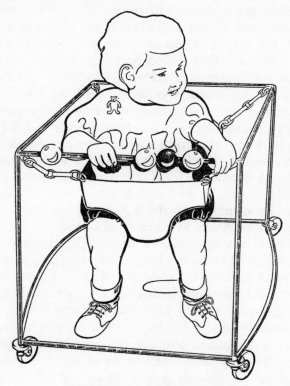

FIGURE 6:1 BABY WALKER

the look of the back, but the maintenance of its structural integrity. In other words, the posture that best protects the disc now takes precedence and the concepts underlying "health-and-beauty" exercises have had to be abandoned. Whereas an endeavour may still be made to correct a child's excessive sway-back, a reasonable hollow at any age is beneficial and to be encouraged.

Prevention should begin in childhood, at home no less than at school. Children should be taught to sit with the back hollowed. Chairs, particularly those attached to a desk, should have a proper back support and the children should be stopped from slouching forwards, and taught to keep their backs against the support. The design of the desk must be such that they can sit this way to read and write—that is, the slope and the height of the working surface must correspond. At gym, no child should be asked to bend forwards, still less to make strenuous efforts to increase the distance down that he can reach. Gymnasts at school must temper their enthusiasm for toe-touching exercises and concentrate instead on the hands-on-hips, knees-bend type, where the knees are used to lower the trunk, which remains upright. All should realise that, the heavier the object to be lifted, the more the back should be hollowed first in order to bear the extra weight safely. A real endeavour should be made to render the maintenance of the hollow in the back second nature, so that everyone, as a matter of course, for the rest of his life, lifts in this way. School medical officers should take pains to ensure that their charges adopt a proper posture while standing and sitting, and, at boarding schools, should make sure that none of the beds sag. At girls' schools, no old-fashioned exercises should be allowed—for example, those that flatten the lumbar spine by drawing the pelvis forwards; for this flexes the lumbar joints from below just as effectively as bending forwards flexes them from above. Complaints of backache in school children should not be ignored, nor should they be regarded as unfounded merely because an X-ray photograph shows that no bone disease is present. When perfectly honest adults are asked when they had their first attack of backache, many of them can remember symptoms starting at the age of perhaps twelve. Children develop imaginary pains, as do adults, but a complaint of backache in adolescence is seldom devoid of organic basis.

Posture in the home

A number of simple precautions can greatly reduce the occasions when spinal flexion is called for in activities around the house. All the household apparatus should be so constructed as to minimise the number of times a housewife needs to bend down. To this end, nothing in daily use should be stacked on the floor or in a low cupboard; such things should be kept on shelves. Sinks and washbasins should be built in much higher than is plumbers' wont. A sneeze while washing the hands, or a cough while brushing the teeth, is a common way to precipitate lumbago; no one should be made to stoop over taps placed too low. Ironing boards are common offenders; they usually need propping up fore and aft on a couple of telephone directories. In the kitchen the working surface for standing at should be some 150 mm (6 inches) higher than the top of the table at which the cook sits.

Every time a housewife bends to lower her hands closer to the floor, she must use her legs, not her back. She should squat to put something into the oven (see Figure 6:2), and go down on one knee and then bend her trunk sideways to get her hand to the floor (see Figure 6:3). An alternative is to stand on one leg, and straighten the other out backwards. The latter keeps her lumbar spine concave, as the trunk swivels at the other hip (see Figure 6:4). Work done on the floor—for example, scrubbing—must be carried out not kneeling, but on all fours (see Figure 6:5). The back is then arched as it hangs between arms and legs; moreover, compression ceases. This is indeed the very position in which the spine originally developed.

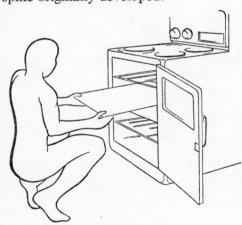

FIGURE 6:2 PUTTING FOOD INTO THE OVEN

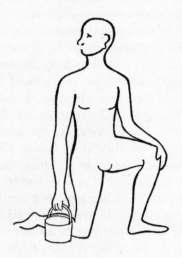

FIGURE 6:3   PICKING UP AN OBJECT FROM THE FLOOR

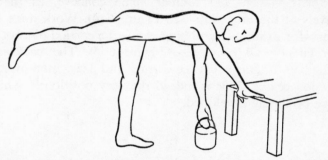

FIGURE 6:4   ALTERNATIVE METHOD OF PICKING UP AN
OBJECT

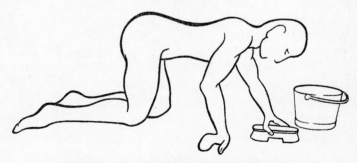

FIGURE 6:5   SCRUBBING THE FLOOR

The chairs round the house should be vetted for a properly shaped back support and fitted with a well-stuffed lumbar cushion if they are wrongly made. Too deep a seat means that the sitter's knees engage against its edge before the spine touches the upright part of the chair. This gap must be filled with a hard cushion. The backs of easy chairs should resemble that shown in Plate 10.

Dressing involves putting socks or stockings on. The individual should sit, supporting the ankle on the thigh just above the knee. The same posture is required for putting on shoes, unless they are loose enough to shuffle into. Laces are best tied by putting the foot on the third or fourth stair and leaning forwards with the back arched until the trunk meets the front of the thigh. The shoe is now within easy reach of the hands (see Figure 6:6).

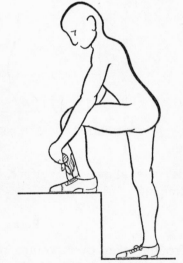

FIGURE 6:6 TYING SHOE LACES

Lying properly in a bath is possible only in shallow water. If it is taken too full, the individual cannot recline and keep his head above water unless the back of his chest is bent well forwards thus losing the lumbar hollow. Not more than 150 mm (6 inches) depth of water enables him to lie flat,

G

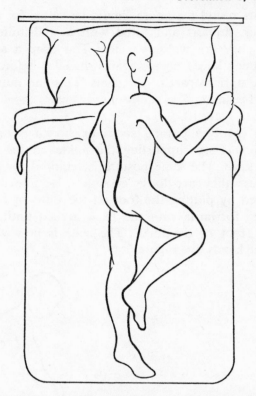

FIGURE 6:7   BEST POSITION FOR LYING IN BED

his nose above the surface, his knees bent and his back straight.

Posture in bed

Trouble taken over posture in bed is good sense; one spends nearly a third of one's life there.

There is nothing worse than the hammock position, which rounds the lumbar spine at each end. It involves flexing the lumbar spine from above, by way of the thoracic joints, and from below, by bending the sacrum forwards as well. There is no way of avoiding this posture, for the recumbent person

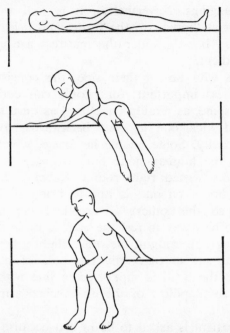

FIGURE 6:8   HOW TO GET OUT OF BED CORRECTLY

has nothing to brace himself against when he tries to restore his lumbar concavity. Admittedly, during lying, the compression stress of weight-bearing no longer acts on the joint; nevertheless, a lot of backache results from sagging mattresses.

Those who habitually lie on their back need a fairly firm mattress, otherwise the hammock posture becomes inevitable, as happens in a feather bed. Those who wake with backache that eases during the day, are probably lying on too soft a mattress—unless they happen to suffer from spondylitis, of which matutinal backache is a common early symptom. A simple test is to put the mattress on the floor and try this out for a few nights. Clearly, if this stops the backache, a harder mattress—often called "orthopaedic"—is required. Young people, as yet with their discs intact, do not bother much what sort of bed is provided for them in, say,

university lodgings. Nevertheless, it is well worth parents'
while to give a thought to the future and insist on one that
does not sag; boards under the mattress are a useful temporary expedient.

For those who lie on their side, the consistency of the
mattress is less important; for people can curl up, flexing
the lumbar spine, as readily on a hard as on a soft mattress.
They should kick one leg out backwards, to restore the
lumbar concavity. Some people lie prone, which is the best
position for the lumbar spine but, in order to breathe, the
neck must be twisted right round. Keeping the neck fully
rotated for hours on end is apt to bring on cervical disc
trouble; hence this otherwise excellent posture is to be
avoided. The best way to rest the back is to lie three-quarters
prone, one leg out straight, the other slightly bent. The chest
is slightly turned so that only one side of it touches the
mattress and the head is supported in line with the thorax,
either on a small pillow or the upstretched arm (see Figure
6:7).

When a patient is asked to lie in bed because of lumbago,
this posture may not prove possible at first, since the back
may be fixed bent forwards. He must then lie in whatever
position relieves pain until the fixation eases, whereupon he
lies flat with a hot water bottle under his lumbar spine, to
induce concavity there. (It is not the heat, which has a
merely comforting effect, but the thickness of the hot water
bottle that does the good.) When the patient first tries to get
out of bed, he should turn on his side and draw up his knees
until the thighs lie at a right angle with his trunk. He now
pushes with his nether arm and brings his body upright
without moving the lumbar joints (see Figure 6:8).

At many clinics in the USA and Canada, it is the custom
to rest patients with lumbago or sciatica in bed with the lower
spine held in flexion. Presumably the idea is to make room
for the displacement thus minimising its effect. Unhappily,
during flexion the back of the joint is more open than the
front, and the tilt of the bony surfaces forces the disc further

backwards towards the dural tube and the nerve root. This posture has, therefore, the opposite effect of that intended (see Figures 1:2 and 1:3).

Reading in bed is difficult during an attack of lumbago, since the usual posture involves flexing the neck and the lumbar spine, unless the book is held in the air by raising the arm vertically. This is too tiring to be kept up for long and a better alternative is to lie prone across the bed, the head projecting over the edge and the book on the floor (see Figure 6:9). An alternative is prismatic spectacles.

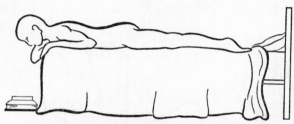

FIGURE 6:9 POSITION FOR READING IN BED DURING LUMBAGO

Making a bed is best carried out kneeling, so that the housewife's hands are kept level with the gap under the mattress where the bedclothes are tucked in.

Childbirth

Lying in bed after a confinement is one of the commonest causes of backache in young women; the attribution comes up time after time. It has nothing to do with the pregnancy and childbirth as such; it is the result of what I have stigmatised as the "nursing mother's posture." The commonest reason for a healthy woman spending ten days in bed is having a baby. She is not ill; she does not want to lie flat; so she is provided with pillows behind her chest and none behind her lumbar spine, which droops into convexity all day. Worse still, she sits up slightly hunched to feed the baby. No woman should lie in bed with one pillow behind her shoulders and another under her knees, leaving the lower back sagging unsupported (see Figure 6:10). She should keep her lower back concave with a thick cushion there and must turn and lie face downwards at intervals during the day, so as to rest the back in the good position (see Figure 6:11). This applies equally to rest in bed for reasons other than childbirth.

Height of the pillow

This should be thick enough to keep the head in the neutral position during recumbency. If the individual normally lies

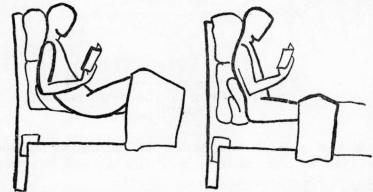

FIGURE 6:10 THE NURSING MOTHER'S POSTURE IN BED
Note the lack of support at the lumbar region which remains flexed all day long. Disc protrusion is thus encouraged

FIGURE 6:11 THE PROPER WAY TO SIT UP IN BED
A special pillow maintains the lumbar concavity, and the posterior longitudinal ligament is spared

on his back, too thick a pillow keeps the neck flexed and in the long run will give him central or bilateral neckache. If he lies on his side, the pillow should be thick enough to occupy the gap between the point of the shoulder and the ear, again keeping the neck in the neutral position.

Posture at night is important in the prevention of stiff necks. Young people are apt to wake up with a stiff neck, having gone to bed comfortable the night before. The cause is lying for hours on end with the head twisted or sideways on. If a loose fragment of disc is present at a joint, keeping the joint-surfaces at considerable angulation for hours on end may well make it slowly shift. On waking, the neck therefore is fixed and painful on one side—a "crick in the neck." In consequence, the sufferer mistakenly regards himself as having slept in a draught. Patients who suffer frequent recurrences must learn to keep their neck as still and as upright as possible, avoiding maintaining the neck bent for long at a time (see Figures 6:12 and 6:13 and Plate 11). If the disorder is apt to come on during the night, a bath towel should be twisted into a rope 15 cm in diameter and worn in bed as a collar. Alternatively, Medisearch's pillow-case is very satisfactory. It converts any ordinary pillow to the correct butterfly shape that supports the head in the neutral position.

No one should sleep on more than one pillow, as two flex the neck excessively. While asleep, moreover, the muscles relax and all the strain falls on the joint.

Posture at the office

Sedentary workers are apt to flex the joints of the neck, the thorax and the lumbar region; hence, trouble at each of these three levels is commonplace.

The person who pores over a book with the neck well bent forward is asking for, and sooner or later will get, central lower neckache spreading to both shoulder-blades. This is especially apt to affect the short-sighted, who are compelled to put their head close to their book. But the situation is easily reversed; the reading matter can be brought up to the eyes. To this end the desk is fitted with a triangle which presents the papers higher up and obliquely to the reader's eyes. He now has to bend his head slightly backwards (see Figure 6: 12). Alternatively, a book can be held in one hand with the elbow at a right-angle supported on the arm of a chair. At the Athenaeum Club in London, in the reading room, stands a remarkable contraption: a pillar of engraved trellis-work brass about 1.25 m (49 inches) high; from this a stand projects on which a book can be placed at eye level in front of the person seated (see Plate 11). The Victorians had never heard of disc-lesions, but they took the correct steps to ensure that the more aristocratic members of society did not have to suffer the pangs of prolonged neck flexion.

Another common disorder amongst those who sit still for too long is the pain at the lower neck and the back of the chest that a secretary develops after sitting typing. She hunches her shoulders and cranes her neck to the left, looking at papers lying horizontally on the table on which her typewriter stands. The remedy is an orchestral music-stand. This is placed straight in front of her, just above the typewriter. She can now keep her head straight and up, bring her shoulders back and stop bending the thoracic extent of her spine (see Figure 6:13).

It is well to realise that the pressure inside the disc is at its greatest during sitting; hence, it really does matter what position is adopted by those who sit a great deal. The way to make this centrifugal force as harmless as possible should be studied. Whenever a man settles into an office chair for continuous work he should force his buttocks backwards as far as they will go, until his lumbar region touches the upright part of the chair. At the level of his lower lumbar spine, some 200 to 250 mm (8 to 10 inches) above the surface of the seat, there should be a lumbar projection. It should be about the thickness of his forearm, and placed where, if he bends his elbow to a right-angle and puts it behind his back, his forearm would then lie. If there is no support here, a cushion, a brief case, or a rolled up coat or towel should be inserted. But sedentary workers must not only be given proper chairs; their work must also be so placed that they can lean back while seated. If a man is poised forwards to look at papers lying horizontally on a desk, it ceases to matter what sort of chair he has been provided with. If he puts his papers on an inclined surface he has to lean backwards to get

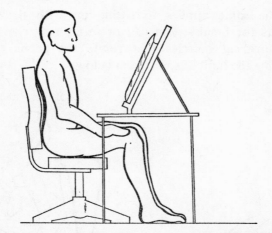

FIGURE 6:12   DESK STAND FOR HOLDING PAPERS

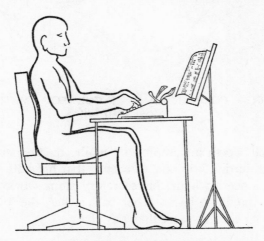

FIGURE 6:13   TYPING DESK AND COPY READING STAND

a good view of them; now his back resumes contact with the lumbar support.

It is unwise to sit with the legs crossed, since the flexion of the uppermost thigh at the hip draws the pelvis forwards, effectively flexing the sacrum on the lumbar spine (see Figure

6:14). The same applies to sitting up with the legs out straight, as for breakfast in bed or in an easy chair; now it is the hamstring muscles that rotate the pelvis forwards, again flexing the lumbar spine from below.

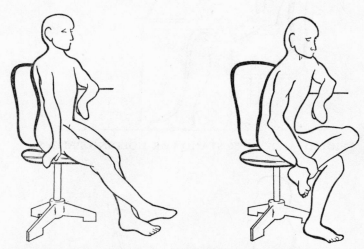

FIGURE 6:14 CORRECT AND INCORRECT METHODS OF CROSSING THE LEGS

It is well worth an employer's while, on financial no less than humanitarian grounds, to ensure that his staff is suitably seated. If, once an hour, his secretary stops work for a few minutes to stand up because her back aches, the lost production has soon cost far more than any chair.

Posture at the factory

A great deal can also be done in a factory. Heavy objects should be presented to workmen at the right height, so that they do not have to stoop. Every man should be taught how to lift. Even if a factory is fully mechanised, with heavy lifting a thing of the past, the man will still lift at home and in his garden, and lumbago brought on during the weekend keeps a man off work just as long. He should bring his hands closer to the ground either by squatting (Figure 6:2), going down on one knee (Figure 6:3), kicking one leg out backwards (see Figure 6:4) or arching his back and letting his hips go, bowing like a flunkey (see Figure 6:15).

Nothing must be lifted with outstretched arms, for this

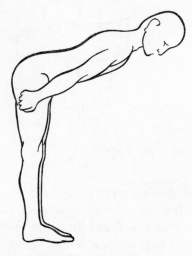

FIGURE 6:15   BENDING FORWARDS—WITH BACK ARCHED

increases leverage. The forward pressure is then increased and the back muscles have to contract considerably harder, thereby compressing the joint much more. Weights should be hugged to the abdomen and if necessary, to the chest, while the knees are being straightened (see Figure 6:16). Just before he lifts, a workman should inhale deeply. As he lifts, he must hold his breath and draw in his abdominal muscles. This manoeuvre produces an upward pressure of chest on abdomen, and some of the weight lifted is borne by pneumatic pressure transferred directly to the pelvis.

A poster on the wall acts as a constant reminder and

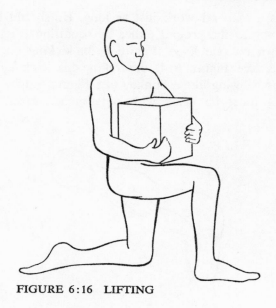

FIGURE 6:16 LIFTING

everyone should receive a posture card to take home (see
Figure 6:17). After all, if only one man out of the whole
labour force is spared a fortnight with lumbago once each
twelve months, any expenditure of less than two weeks' wages
each year would represent a profit. A man caught lifting the
wrong way should be severely reprimanded; for he is want-
only endangering his back and, sooner or later, will defraud
those employing him of wages paid during absence from
work caused by an avoidable industrial accident. If a burden
is carried on on hip, its weight is transmitted to the ground
from the edge of the pelvis to both legs, omitting the lumbar
spine—an excellent plan (see Figure 6:18). Turkish furniture
movers can carry the heaviest pieces by adopting the same
princple; the weight is borne on a saddle applied to the sacrum, so that once more the pressure passes from pelvis to
legs, sparing the back. A rucksack should be given the same
pelvic bearing, the shoulder straps serving merely to balance
the rucksack, not to take its weight.

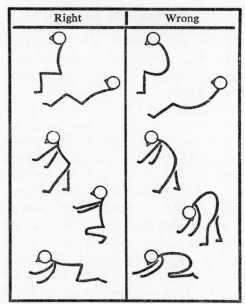

FIGURE 6:17   ST THOMAS'S HOSPITAL POSTURE CHART
This card, showing how to avoid redisplacement in low lumbar disc trouble,
is given to patients

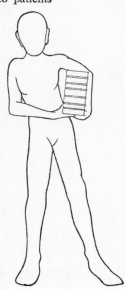

FIGURE 6:18
BALANCING A WEIGHT
ON ONE HIP
If a burden is poised on the
hip bone, its weight is transferred directly to the leg via
the hip joint. No pressure falls
on the lumbar spine

Posture in the garden

The Englishman's well-known love for his garden is responsible for much disc trouble, especially in the lower back. There is probably nothing worse for the lumbar spine than digging, as is evidenced by the standard posture of the gardener in the Victorian illustrations in *Punch*. He stands bent forwards, his hand behind his back, in the typical lumbago position (see Figure 1 : 8). No one should dig. Weeding must be done on all fours. The trouble is that staying in this posture for a long time is very tiring for the arm bearing the weight of the trunk; moreover, only one hand can be used at a time. It is a good idea, therefore, to have a stool with a cushion on it and to lean the chest on that instead.

While raking and hoeing, the implement should be moved by the arms, the body being kept upright. When a wheelbarrow or lawnmower is moved along, the handles should be kept behind the thighs, so that the arms are held slightly backwards arching the trunk (see Figure 6 : 19).

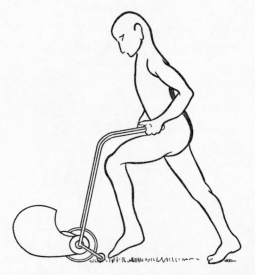

FIGURE 6:19   CORRECT WAY TO MOW THE LAWN

It is unwise to sit in a deckchair. The canvas back describes the arc of a circle and no one thus seated can keep his back hollow. It is better to recline on the lawn on an inflatable mattress.

Posture during sport

Sport enforces certain movements on the performer; he has no choice in the position he has to take up. Moreover, many movements are jerky or complicated by impact with other players. When, therefore, a boy at school develops an early disc-lesion, an awkward situation has to be faced. (He is usually an energetic boy who plays games well and enjoys them; the sluggard does not use any part of his body hard enough to break anything.) On the one hand, he must not be allowed to make his lesion worse; on the other, concern for his back alone must not be allowed to mar his life. The right balance is difficult to achieve.

The only actively beneficial sport is swimming. The swimmer arches his back to keep his head out of the water; moreover, the trunk is floating in a medium of the same specific gravity as itself and all compression strain is obviated. Running and jumping are quite safe.

Rugby football is best avoided, partly because many discs are first cracked by a kick in the small of the back, partly because the scrum entails strong compression of the lumbar spine while it is held flexed. If a boy is really keen, he can try playing and see what happens, but only out of the scrum. The scrum is also responsible for much initial damage to the discs in the neck. While the players are locked shoulder to shoulder, the head is kept out of the way by full neck flexion. Any sideways jar to the neck as the players move catches the cervical joints in their most vulnerable position and many stiff necks originate this way.

Rowing involves full forward bending at the lumbar joints and must be avoided once a disc-lesion has developed there. Riding is harmless as long as the patient does not tire. While he is fresh, he uses his muscles to keep his back hollow—the correct seat. If he tires, he may slump, reversing the curve of his back; hence he must stop short of fatigue or wear a corset, as did the Austrian cavalry officer early this century.

Golf seldom affects a lumbar disc-lesion but, of course, the player must bend his knees to pick the ball out of the hole, and when putting should not stay bent forwards for too long. Patients who have thoracic disc trouble must avoid so great a follow through when driving that the extreme of rotation of the trunk is reached. Such straining of the joint is apt to bring on the pain at the back of the chest—and sometimes lumbar pain too—which can be avoided if the twisting movement is brought to a slightly earlier halt.

Posture while travelling

Falling asleep while upright in a train means that the neck falls into flexion while the muscles are relaxed. This is a common cause of a painful stiff neck in young people who cannot afford a sleeper.

When luggage is carried, it is as well to remember that two suitcases weighing, say, 10 kg (22 lb) each compress the spinal joints by 20 kg (44 lb). By contrast, one suitcase weighing 20 kg (44 lb) carried in one hand forces the muscles to mount an equal counter-pressure on the other side of the body to stop it tilting over. The consequent compression strain is therefore 40 kg. Whatever is carried, the arm should be brought behind the centre of gravity of the body, so that the traction force on it brings the trunk slightly backwards (see Figure 6:20).

A great deal of sitting goes on in cars, trains and aeroplanes. In European trains, anyone who is not exceptionally tall does better to travel in a second- rather than a first-class compartment, where the seats are deeper. If the seat is longer than the distance from the back of his knees to the convexity of his buttocks, the traveller cannot apply his lower trunk against the upright part of the seat. Hence, unless he has brought a support with him, he is forced to sit with his lumbar spine convex. In an aeroplane, a briefcase is useful to sit against, or the air-hostess can be asked for a small blanket, which is rolled up and put some 200 mm (8 inches) above the horizontal part of the seat.

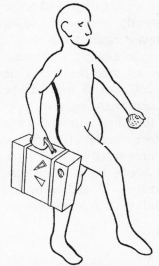

FIGURE 6:20   CARRYING A SUITCASE

Car seats

These cause so much trouble that they merit separate consideration. A very common complaint is that of such discomfort that the driver has to get out for five minutes each hour to rid himself of increasing backache. After a few minutes' standing, the pain goes—that is, restoring the concavity to the lower back encourages the nuclear bulge to recede. Had he sat with his back properly supported in the hollow position, the ache would not have come on. The number of back rests offered for sale to motorists bears witness to the bad design of most car seats today. It costs no more to make an anatomical seat than one that ignores the shape of the body; yet my twenty-five years of homilies in medical and motoring journals have had scarcely any effect.

H

Bad design is also apparent in pilots' seats in military and civil aircraft.

If a car seat is too low, the driver's legs are held nearly straight. In this position, the hamstring muscles pull the lower pelvis forwards, thus flexing the lumbar spine from below. A minimum angle between thigh and lower leg is 30 degrees. If a car seat is strictly horizontal, nothing encourages the driver's back to engage against the vertical part of the seat. It should, therefore, be slightly tilted and the upper surface should be slippery, so that the thighs do slide backwards. Just about 200 to 250 mm (8 to 10 inches) above the horizontal part of the seat is the support, approximately 80 mm (3¼ inches) wide, that fits into and maintains the driver's lumbar concavity (see Figure 6:21). It comes exactly where an individual's forearm rests when he puts it horizontally behind his back. It should be held in position by two short vertical bars, so that it can be slid up or down a small distance and fixed there to suit each separate driver.

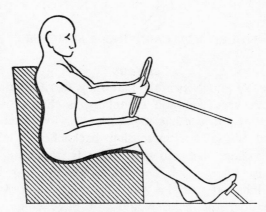

FIGURE 6:21   IDEAL CAR SEAT
Tilted car seat with further inclination to accommodate buttocks; head-rest
is not shown

In the car, a head-rest fixed to the car seat prevents the head being shot backwards on unforeseen impact from behind, sometimes resulting in a whiplash injury to the neck (see page 32).

Good-natured people often help to push a broken-down car off the road. The safe way to do this is to apply the buttocks to the back of the car and push it with one's legs (see Figure 6:22).

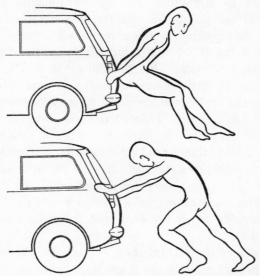

FIGURE 6:22   CORRECT AND INCORRECT WAYS TO PUSH A CAR

Postural exercises

It is an accepted orthopaedic principle that the stronger the muscles are about a joint, the more stable it is. In general, this is true, and a strong muscle spanning a joint, as it runs from one bone to another, is clearly an advantage. But who puts the cartilage out in his knee? The professional foot-baller's exceptionally strong muscles enable him to put strains on the joint that an ordinary person cannot. Since there is no muscle running from the bone to the cartilage, the power-ful muscle is now of no help. In fact, at the spinal joints it is the ligaments and the interdigitation of the bony facets that ensure stability (see Figure 3:1); the muscles merely first compress, then move, the joints between the vertebrae. Compression sets up centrifugal force, so this is no advantage, to say the least, and the man whose strong muscles enable him to lift, say, 100 kg is applying more compression than his weaker brother who can lift only 50 kg.

Exercises to strengthen the lumbar muscles are entirely valueless. However, all this century, patients, doctors, physiotherapists and gymnasts have remained certain that backache is the result of weak lumbar muscles, and that *the* treatment is exercises. This orthodoxy is so ingrained that consideration of basic principles seems to have been omitted; hence, the futility of the ordinary type of postural exercises is still not recognised. Indeed, doctors tend to dismiss as fanciful, or prompted by laziness, patients' complaints that exercises make their backache worse. Nevertheless, the patients are right; postural exercises *are* harmful in backache.

There is only one beneficial exercise in back troubles: to inculcate the maintenance of a constant postural tone in the lumbar muscles so as to keep the joint motionless in the good position.

If the disc has cracked, but is fully in place, the loose fragment cannot move again if the joint is never moved again. The use, then, of muscle contraction to prevent the joint moving is a clear advantage; whereas, if it is used to move the joint, another opportunity for displacement is created. It is, of course, an exercise for the muscles when they keep the joint still against stress tending to move it, but this is not what patients understand by exercises, which to them involve moving both joint and muscles together. Exercises bending forwards are the most harmful, and the ordinary exercise that most patients are taught—lying prone and lifting head and legs backwards—is less harmful; but doing no exercises at all is better still. The correct aim is to maintain a slight contraction the whole time so as to keep the joint always as motionless as possible in the safe position.

Transatlantic readers will note that the facts set out here conflict strongly with the considerations underlying what are known in the United States as "Williams's exercises," and in Canada as "Goldthwaite's exercises." Both, in my view, should be assiduously avoided.

Exercising machines

All sorts of machines are advocated by their manufacturers largely for slimming, and, of course, any exercise of any sort has this effect. Those that tense (not stretch) the abdominal muscles possess the advantage of selectively strengthening them.

Nearly all these contraptions are designed with little thought for the joints of the spine, and quite a few involve trunk flexion. Some require postures that could easily injure a lumbar disc or cause displacement of one already damaged.

Prospective purchasers would do well to consider critically the postures involved.

Watkin's guide

My colleague Dr B. Watkin has kindly contributed a guide for motorists wishing to avoid, or already liable to, backache. He has tested all these car seats himself and has declared his assessment on the guide-book principle of awarding asterisks—see Appendix.

7

Economics of Disc Trouble

There is no doubt in my mind that the commonest cause of *avoidable* absence from work is disc trouble. Sooner or later every worker faces the economic effects of a slipped disc, so does the employer himself, both personally and in regard to the proper running of his business by his men.

Doctors are interested in patients, nor their finances, and the economic effect of different ways of treating disease hardly impinges on medical ways of thought. Little attention is paid to the different economic results of various methods of treatment; the doctor's concern is to get his patient well without much regard for the time factor. When it is a question of life and death, or the prevention of severe crippledom, cost is immaterial. Hence, a disorder that proffers no threat to life, but merely to livelihood, is apt to be regarded with some detachment by medical men. Patients too; for they are angered rather than alarmed at their predicament—quite correctly.

The example of lumbago and sciatica

At the turn of the century, lumbago was thought of as "fibro-sitis" and mistaken for a disease of muscle because the pain was felt in the muscles. In those days, this error made treatment for the muscles by rest, heat and massage appear logical; it was based on a mistake, but was a perfectly reasonable extension from this basis. Now, my attribution of lumbago to a deranged joint is largely accepted, but for reasons obscure to me, treatment by rest in bed, heat, massage and exercises is still widely practised. Recumbency much diminishes the pressure on the joint, and lying flat eventually stops the flexion in which the joint is fixed. In consequence, the loose fragment slowly retraces its steps; after two to four weeks the patient has recovered and is fit for work again. But there is another way of treating lumbago: manipulating the loose piece back into place. Our figures (Barbor, 1955) show that 53 per cent of patients thus treated go back to work the next day. Indeed, all doctors—and most people, too—are acquainted with patients who, after many fruitless weeks in bed under the best auspices, have visited a lay manipulator and been put right on the spot. This situation is common knowledge and was criticised in *The Times* by Philip Noel-Baker MP (1963).

The economic result of this changed concept, therefore, has so far proved negligible. This gap in medical services has led to patients going behind their doctor's back to lay manipulators, hoping to be made well faster. This laudable endeavour sometimes succeeds, sometimes fails; for it is only the doctor, after a full medical examination, who can tell whether manipulation is likely to prove effective or not. Everyone would benefit, therefore, if this state of affairs were brought out into the open. In the meanwhile, the manager of a large firm, anxious to resume charge at his office, is still expected to moulder in bed awaiting spontaneous recovery from a disorder that is, in fact, often relievable there and then. He is also compelled to accept the same costly delay among his employees. Both he and his men suffer needlessly, as they did in past centuries before the mechanism of lumbago was elucidated. The logical implementation of this change in concept has sadly lagged behind. Now that lumbago is widely acknowledged as due to a displacement within the joint, it would seem reasonable that

the first thought in treatment would be concern to move it
back into position again. Why does passive resignation still
obtrude in the management of these cases? It is surely time
that the doctors of the world and their patients got together
to insist that active treatment for such a common disorder
should be made available at every hospital. Every physiotherapy department should contain at least one member of
staff trained in spinal manipulation. To a limited extent,
the public has already taken the treatment of lumbago into
its own hands. Many executives, having discovered for
themselves how greatly lay manipulators can sometimes ex-
pedite recovery, insist on valued employees doing the same.
Hence, private enterprise has taken over from the medical
profession and to some extent conceals the gap.

Elementary but unarguable economics

It is true that the result of treating lumbago with bed-rest
and manipulation is the same—in the end. After, say, a month
has elapsed, patients who have undergone either treatment
are well, and the medical attitude is congratulatory. However, the long-term patient has got well at financial loss:
to himself if he is self-employed, or to industry if he
is salaried; and, in either event, the nation has sustained a
loss.

Let us leave the humanitarian aspect to one side and consider finance only. If a man earning £100 a week has been
off work for four weeks, he has received £400 for nothing.
If a manipulation costing £10 as a private patient puts him
right after a day or two, £350 or more has been saved.
Patients attending a hospital out-patient clinic cost the British
hospital service about £1 a head. Were the patient earning
only £20 a week, and one manipulation was successful, it
would be a matter of one day's absence (cost £4+£1) against
one month's absence viz: £80). But that is only one side
of the situation. When suitable out-patient measures are not
available, many patients are perforce admitted to hospital.

This is a positive expense to be added to the negative loss. A bed in hospital costs the State £25 to £60 a week. Hence, in many instances another, say, £80 per patient is expended needlessly. I am convinced that arrangements for the provision of a remedy, already widely known often to be quick and effective, would save at least a hundred times the outlay.

Any employer can find this out for himself. If he has a large factory at which, at any one time, say, ten men earning £40 a week are expected to be off work for four weeks, and adequate treatment enables half to return to work after only one day's absence, he has saved his firm £150 a month five times over—that is, £750 less the cost of the physiotherapist. A physiotherapist's salary is about £150 a month. If the employer appointed to his staff one expert in manipulation, who saw a mere two patients a day, he would save himself four times her annual salary every month. This does not take into consideration other large gains from treating stiff necks, painful shoulders, sprained knees and so on, that also obtain speedy relief from accurate, but largely unobtainable, manual treatment.

A doctor skilled in the methods of orthopaedic medicine has not much difficulty in seeing twenty patients a day. If he works a five-day week at a salary of £10 000 a year (which would be considered quite generous in the UK) each patient would cost £2. He could not fail, by treating the diseases of the moving parts that keep so many men off work (each for some weeks), every month to save the firm employing him his yearly salary. This is a very conservative estimate. It therefore surprises me that there exists no large concern in the country that is eager to employ such a doctor or a trained physiotherapist. It is obvious that this would be the case if industry were aware that doctors exist who can deal with the problem and that physiotherapists also exist who, given a chance, would cope. There is no secret about these facts. As long ago as 1956, the medical officer attached to Arthur Guinness, Son and Company Limited in Dublin published a paper describing the result in cases of lumbago of sending two of his physiotherapists to St Thomas's Hospital for a mere fortnight's tuition (Pringle, 1956). I know that many large firms do possess a physiotherapy department, but in most cases it is largely devoted to the provision of diathermy, massage and exercises for disorders that derive little benefit from such measures.

The manner of accounting makes a big difference. Dr Hirschfeld of Bremen came over to England some ten years ago and took the methods of orthopaedic medicine (and one of my best physiotherapy graduates) back to Germany with him. After a year, the actuary of the Health Service there had noticed the greatly enhanced speed of recovery in patients seen by him, compared to statistics based on previous years' invalidism. At the end of another year, the superiority of orthopaedic medicine over traditional methods remained clear. As a result, a hospital department was built for Hirschfeld and a lesser premium offered to employers if they would agree that their workmen, if unable to work for an orthopaedic medical reason, should go to his department only. In Germany, his work attracted favourable attention within a year, since the system there is based on cost per patient. Hence, the spectacular diminution in time off work, in sick pay and in doctors' fees drew immediate attention to itself.

In 1963, one of my hospital colleagues published a paper on the treatment of severe sciatica, using an injection that I had sponsored for over thirty years, comparing it with recumbency. It turned out that one or two injections had the same effect in ten days, the patient resting at home, as was secured by admission to hospital for pure rest in bed for thirty days. As in-patients at a teaching hospital in Britain cost more than £50 a week, it was a question of £2 as against £220. Moreover, the injection was shown to be three times quicker, and a hospital bed was liberated and therefore ready for occupancy by some other sufferer. It might have been thought that this telling piece of controlled research, published in the *British Medical Journal*, would have been followed by widespread adoption, or at least trial, of this injection. It was not.

The cost to the UK

Progress in medicine has been such that many of the scourges of the early part of this century are half forgotten. Tuberculosis, pneumonia and diphtheria no longer take an appreciable toll. Advances in medicine and surgery have been so great that many once-common and serious disorders have ceased to endanger us appreciably (see Figure 7:1). As a drain on the nation's purse, however, their place has been taken by disorders less emotionally charged, not threatening life or limb, but industrially just as disabling. As a result, though large numbers of patients no longer die or spend months off work with pneumonia and its aftermath, the period of invalidism caused by lumbago, for example, has not changed. This fact has not led to the provision of funds for the dissemination of knowledge of how such conditions are best managed, since the feeling engendered by locomotor disorders is not strong enough to evoke donations from the public or from industry. Nevertheless, it is here where money would be so well spent, not so much on research (for that has been largely completed), but on the application of treatments already in existence on a scale large enough to cover the whole country.

Data derived from a study of 6.5 million periods of absence from work were put forward at a symposium held in Glasgow in 1966. The analysis showed that 5.1 per cent of all absence in men, and 2.4 per cent in women, were due to back troubles. In figures for those drawing injury, not sickness, benefit, the proportions rose to 11.4 per cent in men and 6.2 per cent in women. Remarkable figures emerged for the average length of time off work with back troubles. Sciatica (which, after all, can last some time) accounted for only 13 per cent of these patients. Yet the average periods of disablement for backache turned out to be 13 weeks in men

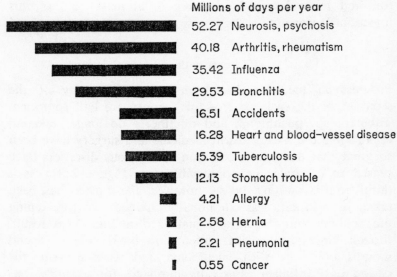

	Millions of days per year
	52.27 Neurosis, psychosis
	40.18 Arthritis, rheumatism
	35.42 Influenza
	29.53 Bronchitis
	16.51 Accidents
	16.28 Heart and blood-vessel disease
	15.39 Tuberculosis
	12.13 Stomach trouble
	4.21 Allergy
	2.58 Hernia
	2.21 Pneumonia
	0.55 Cancer

FIGURE 7:1   GRAPH OF FREQUENCY OF ABSENCE FROM WORK
IN BRITAIN FOR VARIOUS ILLNESSES

and 17 weeks in women under 25 years old. After the age
of 45, these periods rose to 22 and 24 weeks respectively.
Since there must be many reasonable people in Glasgow who
return to work after the ordinary absence of a few weeks,
these averages indicate that many people are taking a year
off for lumbago. If these long periods of idleness are
countenanced over large parts of Britain, and in any way
represent the general situation, a medical service orientated
towards the moving parts of the body (what I call
"orthopaedic medicine") would pay handsome dividends
indeed.

Many of these patients that have been described are
anxious to get well. Others are in less of a hurry, but are
prepared to admit that they are pain-free once they have
recovered. Yet no one really caters adequately for this important mass of people with locomotor troubles. They wander
from doctor to doctor, then from hospital to hospital, hoping
to find an interested medical man. Many despair and, on

their friends' advice, start to frequent lay manipulators. This search for relief is on their own initiative, at their own expense; not from foolishness, but from lack of anywhere near adequate facilities and medico-physiotherapeutic personnel to deal with such lesions of the moving parts.

The number of manipulating laymen, and their undoubted successes, together with the esteem which many members of the public accord them, indicates the large number of patients who have been driven to visit them. However, account must also be taken of the waste of time and money involved in treatment without proper diagnosis. Accurate diagnosis cannot be expected of individuals who have not undergone a full medical training. Hence, interspersed with the successes, are those cases where recourse to laymen leads to much prolonged, expensive and futile treatment for conditions that manipulation cannot effect. Even if the patient has a slipped disc, only about half of all cases benefit from manipulation. Throughout, it is the patient who bears the diagnostic onus of deciding that manipulation is necessary; the layman merely carries it out. Each individual has to take his chance with anyone in his district who holds himself out as a manipulator, whether or not he has had any training.

It is a fact that the industrial efficiency of Britain is in part maintained by a series of self-styled manipulators whom each individual has to select without medical guidance, not knowing whether his trouble is likely to respond to such treatment, nor where to find a trained person. In Britain today, the ordinary member of the public has no means of distinguishing those lay manipulators who have had some training from those—the majority—who have had none. It is true that the letters MRO (Member of the Register of Osteopaths) after a man's name cannot be assumed by the unrecognised, but how is the potential patient to know that? The problem is not small nor unimportant.

The overall cost of National Insurance claims to the nation in 1965 was summarised in the *British Medical Journal* of 8 January 1966.

Nearly 21 million people in Great Britain are covered by National Insurance sickness benefit. They make about 9 million claims a year and lose about 300 million working days through notified incapacity—that is spells of four days or more. Bronchitis accounts for nearly 40 million of these days, arthritis and rheumatism for 20 million, and psychoses and psychoneuroses for 27 million. The annual cost in National Insurance is over £220 million.

The Industrial Survey Unit of the Arthritis and Rheumatism Council conducted a ten-year survey, which reported in 1969. They worked out that the financial burden on industry from this cause amounted to £150 million in wages alone. They considered that many more millions were lost from disruption of work and diminished productivity. Absence because of locomotor disease proved highest in work involving awkward positions, exerting the back or lifting weights. Dockers and miners headed the statistics with 373 days a year for each 100 men at risk. (It must be remembered that the figures for sickness by far exceed loss of work from strikes.) These figures include rheumatic disorders other than disclesions. A Swedish doctor published figures based on a survey of 62 000 cases of locomotor trouble that suggest that half of all disease ascribed to rheumatism is, in fact, caused by disc-lesions.

Neurosis

Then there is the question of neurosis. Neurosis is uncommon after fractures and after injuries sustained at home or during sport, whereas after car smashes or accidents at work emotional reactions are apt to follow since claims for compensation then arise. Even so, the patient who suffers an accident, say to his back, at work is unlikely to develop neurosis if he is dealt with quickly and competently. Clearly, if he has a displaced fragment of disc and it is put back that day or the next, whereupon he resumes work, he has neither time nor inclination for emotional upset.

By contrast, he may find himself lying in bed for a week or two without improving much. Despondent at his lack of progress and coming gradually round to the understandable idea that, since nothing *is* being done for him, nothing *can* be done, he considers his future as a disabled man, and remembers that the cause was an accident at work. He consults his solicitor and traumatic neurasthenia begins to take hold. It is kept in being by the anxieties and delays of litigation. The cases that come to court are seldom settled in less than three or four years. During the whole of this time, the patient has to lend colour to his claims by staying off work. This means financial loss, and now his worries become better founded. Medico-legal negotiations continue. These are not concerned with getting the patient well, but are a compromise between the solicitor's endeavour to get full justice for his client and an attempt to reconcile various doctors' views on what is the matter with him, whether he will recover fully or not, and how long this may take. The wretched patient who was earning, say, £1000 a year, after four years of idleness may receive £1000 or £2000 compensation but he stands a fair chance of losing his suit and getting nothing. The characteristics of neurosis are fully described in the next chapter. Quite good prevention of this type of trouble is to explain to him that even if he wins his case, he loses financially. The best prophylaxis is prompt treatment.

Doctors and patients are both well aware of this situation. Insurance companies and the officials administering sickness benefit must be perturbed. The medical officers of large firms doubtless report their concern to their boards of directors, but so far have not hit on the remedy; for many are unaware of the benefits that orthopaedic medicine offers. All these powerful institutions, facing a recurrent and long-standing problem in which finance and the relief of human suffering both point in the same direction, have proved impotent to overcome widespread inertia. So have I.

8

Neurosis and Litigation

Neurosis is conspicuously rare after injuries incurred at home, or during games or sport. It seldom follows fractures since these are detected at once by X-ray examination and are dealt with promptly and effectively. Neurosis is apt to supervene, as was pointed out in the last chapter, after an injury sustained at work or in a car crash as, in both these instances, the question of compensation arises.

In Britain, one potent factor in provoking neurosis is the traditional treatment of disc-lesions, which is also unwittingly calculated to engender anxiety. Indeed, it is a tribute to the stolidity and goodwill of the people in this country that there are not more cases of neurosis. A simple example, familiar to every employer, is as follows. A workman lifts a heavy weight and is stricken by a severe pain in his back. He can scarcely move and, after lying down for a while, is taken home and put to bed. His doctor visits him and tells him perhaps that he has lumbago, or perhaps that he has a slipped disc. This is correct, for they are different names for the same entity. Many patients recover in a few weeks, but the occasional case recovers spontaneously only after some months. In the latter event, he lies in bed day after day, not getting much better, so he is sent up to hospital by ambulance, X-rayed and seen by a doctor there, told that no serious disease is detectable, assured that he has nothing to worry about and enjoined further rest in bed. After another week or two of recumbency has brought only slight relief, the patient, understandably enough, begins to become anxious about himself and his future. "Reassurance that no crippling disorder is present," he says to himself, "is all very well, but have I got a condition for which no treatment exists? If there were any treatment, surely by now I should be getting it? Anyhow, if I cannot go to work, that in itself is serious to me, if not to doctors, in the economic sense. If my state really cannot be relieved, I may well never be fit for heavy work again. How then," he broods, "am I to earn my living in the future?" Introspection increases, not without reason, and he now remembers that the cause was an incident at work. Ideas of compensation for the apparently irremediable injury begin to burgeon. He discusses the matter with his friends, who shake their heads and regale him with tales of their relations' disc troubles, which have ended, perhaps, in operation or permanent disablement. Alarmed, he sends for his solicitor and is thenceforward caught up in toils from which he cannot escape.

Contrast that sorry sequence with that of the same man who suffers the same injury, is visited by his doctor the same day, manipulated or given an epidural injection the same day, and is seen again the following day. He is re-examined and treated anew, if necessary, according to the findings present then. He feels himself in brisk and capable hands; he finds the treatment effective and within a few days is back at work.

The first man, once enmeshed with the law can no longer afford to recover. As his backache slowly eases and finally ceases, so do his months off work accumulate and increasingly compel him to go on seeking compensation. This mounts up only if his disablement continues. The original backache, now gone, is replaced by what is variously termed "traumatic"— that is, due to an injury—or "compensation" neurasthenia.

I

Compensation neurasthenia

This term is applied to neurosis following an accident from which recovery has ensued, but the notion of disordered function persists, kept in being by the anxieties attendant on impending litigation. It is an interesting fact that in France and eastern European countries, where compensation is obtainable for bodily injury but no account is taken of emotional attitudes, neurasthenia after an accident is virtually unknown. Neurasthenia is a self-engendered disorder, kept in being by a wish to make the most of the accident long after its effects have passed off, and aggravated by the delays and anxieties of litigation.

In the UK, cases seldom reach the courts less than four years after the accident. During the whole of this time, the patient has to lend colour to his story by keeping off work, even such work as he could, by his own admission, undertake. He pesters his doctor. Moreover, solicitors like their client to be receiving "hospital treatment," since this adds weight to the allegation of disablement. Hence, he insists on being sent to the nearest clinic, where he exasperates the physiotherapist by his stubborn refusal to get any better or to discontinue attendance. Rightly, she feels that her efforts are vain: a situation she comes to resent. This sequence leads to irritation all round. Continued unemployment involves further financial loss and leads to worry about chances of eventual reimbursement.

The patient's anxiety now becomes well-grounded and is augmented by the strains of protracted negotiation. These negotiations, unhappily, are no longer concerned with how best to speed his recovery, but with repeated medico-legal examinations, reconciling contradictory opinions on what is the matter with him, how long it may be before he recovers, how much permanent disablement may ensue, and how much monetary compensation he deserves. By now, his preoccupations have become very real, though they have become (like everyone else's concerned with his case) centred on the probable result of litigation.

In the end, the patient's neurasthenia begins to develop a factual basis. The prospect of another medical examination in six months' time, then another, equally inconclusive, after that, causes real anxiety and is also calculated to engender an exasperation that leads him to wish for an agreed settlement rather than an expensive court case of uncertain outcome. If this does not prove so, the doctor's efforts to prevent the case from dragging on from year to year usually prove futile and, in those with a less stable attitude to life, lasting emotional tension may ensue.

Examination in suspected compensation neurosis

Patients with pain devoid of factual basis naturally gravitate to the orthopaedic physician, since in his normal work he deals so largely with patients whose symptoms give rise to few or no objective signs. If the patient is examined by the methods of orthopaedic medicine it is difficult for imagined disorders to escape detection, or at least to arouse strong suspicion, at the first attendance. On the one hand, it is no substitute for diagnosis to regard every patient with symptoms whose cause is not immediately apparent as suffering from neurosis; on the other hand, equal confusion arises from too ready an acceptance of patients' allegations. The physician must maintain the difficult balance between excessive scepticism and over-kindly credulity. Obviously, nervous people are just as likely to develop disc-lesions as anyone else. The difference lies in their reaction to their discomfort. A pain that would merely annoy an ordinary individual may be interpreted by a patient in a state of high tension as severe, or as indicating an important disease, like cancer. In consequence, he may be largely disabled by a pain that another person would shrug off. Nevertheless, before the pain started, he could cope. He had lived a useful life, working well and managing despite his neurosis for years, until this added burden threw him off his balance. In these cases, the proper approach is to get rid of the symptoms on which rests the whole edifice of apprehension. He is treated in the ordinary way, merely with allowance for his hypersensitivity.

Difficult cases are those that I label "half-and-half." The patient does have minor discomfort occasionally, but prefers to harp on it and to remain disabled beyond reason. These individuals usually benefit more from psychological treatment than from anything done to their spine, but sometimes a combined approach is rewarding. It is when a patient's pain has no organic basis at all that the difficult problem arises of altering the circumstances that have given rise to the emotional reaction. Patients do not always like to have their escape from reality blocked; hence, this endeavour is not always successful.

The doctor who concentrates on the non-surgical disorders of the moving parts is in a strong position when the question of neurosis arises. He treads on firm ground, whereas the doctor who is confronted with a possible neurotic cause for headache or indigestion can only surmise that this is so by summing up the patient after every test for organic trouble has proved negative. But the moving parts visibly perform known functions in a known manner. They are thus easy to test. Therefore, the diagnosis of neurosis no longer rests on suppositions with a negative basis, but on the discovery of positive inconsistencies. The self-contradictory findings in these cases are nearly always multiple, and, given enough opportunity, the patient himself soon declares his own insincerity.

Patients with genuine trouble, however many movements are tested, give responses that are consistent with each other and are referable to one anatomical structure. They do not have to answer at random, whereas the neurotic has to guess at the proper answer, and gets it wrong. Inconsistencies are:

1   Between the patient's appearance and his degree
     of suffering

2 Between his symptoms and his posture and gait
3 Between his symptoms, even accepted at his own valuation, and the degree of his disablement
4 Between the site of pain originally and where it has spread to since
5 Between the site of pain and the movements stated to increase it
6 Between what he says he cannot do and the signs found present on examination
7 Between one set of signs at one part of the body and another set of signs elsewhere
8 Between the range of painfulness of a movement carried out one way and then repeated in a different way
9 Between a limited range of movement in one direction and what is found when the joint is tested in other directions
10 Between the size of a muscle belly and allegations of weakness
11 Between the signs proffered and the place alleged to be tender to the touch
12 Between the site of tenderness at one moment and then at another.

There is one apparent inconsistency against which doctors must be warned. It is often maintained that if trunk-flexion is restricted by pain in the back, straight-leg raising must be limited too, and that a discrepancy is evidence of ill-faith. This is not so. The converse does hold; if straight-leg raising is limited, the capacity to bend forwards must be limited too. But, when a patient stands, his body weight compresses the disc so that the protrusion becomes maximal. Lying down, compression ceases and the protrusion tends to recede slightly. This removes the bar to full straight-leg raising. In consequence, many perfectly sincere patients with not very severe lumbago cannot bend forwards but possess a full range of straight-leg raising.

Prevention of neurosis

Immediate treatment

Neurasthenia has no time or reason to develop when immediate and effective treatment is combined with a clear statement of the nature and expected course of the disorder present. This applies particularly to disc-lesions.

Financial advice

During the early days, the plaintiff does not realise how long the time lag is before the case reaches the courts. My first endeavour in the disposal of these cases is, therefore, to explain the financial position to the patient. He is paid, let us say, £3000 a year. By remaining off work for probably five years, he will receive about £4000 in sickness benefit. If he is lucky enough to win his case, he will get perhaps £2000, and he stands about an even chance of a favourable verdict. He cannot, therefore, lose less than £9000, and stands an equal chance of losing another £2000 as well. He would do better for himself to jettison his legal advisers, abandon the suit, swallow his pride and return to work. If he agrees to this policy, I order him a fortnight's "treatment" so that he can allege, without loss of face, that a miraculous cure has taken place.

Treatment

This consists of encouraging the patient to accept a reasonable sum and to return to work. Unfortunately, this is just what his legal advisers may not countenance; for it is their duty to accept his complaints at their face value and to ensure his getting his apparent deserts to the full.

All treatment until the case is settled is vain, though the patient seeks it persistently on his solicitor's advice. If he insists, I see him again and examine him again at as protracted intervals as he will allow me. However long he cares to keep coming, he is given a patient hearing, another examination and *no* treatment. In consequence, the plaintiff,

I feel sure, goes off in the end to some other hospital and tries his luck there.

Malingering

Unfortunately, no way exists for a medical man to draw an objective distinction between neurosis, hysteria and malingering. The manifold inconsistencies that demonstrate the absence of organic disease and the presence of emotionally determined symptoms are present and are the same in all three disorders. If the patient is regarded as possessing an unconscious belief in his condition, neurosis is diagnosed. If the disability depends on such (mistaken) conviction that some part of the body has become functionless, that he allows it to be paralysed or held fixed, the term hysteria is often applied. If the patient knows his symptoms to be assumed, he is a malingerer. But no objective method of assessment has yet been devised, and one doctor may use one label, another another, depending on his sympathy or lack of it with each individual. This difficulty can be resolved only when it becomes possible for a doctor to see into a patient's mind and determine whether a mistaken idea is wilfully or unconsciously maintained.

This is a very tiresome limitation to medical knowledge for employers, barristers and judges to have to face, but there it is.

Laymen's negligence and fees

The dissatisfied client of a layman cannot contest a request for payment for treatment merely by sheltering behind allegations of lack of official recognition, of experience or of competence. No particular standard of knowledge and expertise can be legally enjoined upon unqualified persons. This was decided by the courts in the case of Sones *v* Foster, reported in *The Times* on 21 January 1937. It was held that the defendant, a naturopath, even when giving medical treatment, could be expected to possess "merely the knowledge of the body to which he belonged." The patient makes his own decision, and receives the layman's attentions at his own risk. By contrast, a doctor is tacitly understood, and legally bound, to bring to the patient the degree of skill and conscientious care that is universally expected of a medical man. This duty is not imposed on laymen. When a bonesetter is visited, all that is taken for granted between him and his client is that some part of him will be manipulated. Hence if harm results from such manoeuvres, his client must expect considerable difficulty in proving negligence and securing compensation, since there is no agreed criterion of what amount of knowledge a lay manipulator can be expected to possess. From doctors, patients receive an informed opinion on which subsequent action is based, from a bonesetter the patient requests and receives a manipulation. If this proves injurious, whose fault is that?

The British law governing legal action to secure payment of fees by medically unqualified persons is contained in section 27 of the Medical Act 1956.

> No person shall be entitled to recover any charge
> in any court of law for any medical or surgical
> advice or attendance, or for the performance of
> any operation, or for any medicine which he shall
> have both prescribed and supplied, unless he shall
> prove upon the trial that he is fully registered.

This section implies that an action can be brought against the debtor only if the practitioner was medically fully qualified at the time when the services in question were rendered. The unqualified manipulator is not debarred from suing for work done short of a surgical operation—for example, the administration of heat, exercises, massage and manipulation. But he is debarred from entering a claim for giving the advice on which the choice of treatment rested. Hence, in cases where both advice and treatment are given, he must separate the amounts and sue for the fraction arising from treatment only. In fact, lay manipulators scarcely ever sue for fees, since they do not wish for publicity for their disgruntled patients' statements.

A physiotherapist treats patients only at a doctor's request. He gives the advice; she gives the treatment. Hence her entire bill must be met.

Barristers' guide

In the course of a lawsuit, doctors engaged by the two opposing sides often offer quite different opinions in a case of alleged disc-lesion. Naturally, both judge and counsel prefer to base their views on what they consider to be ascertainable fact—that is, on the radiographic appearances—rather than on clinical evidence. As an X-ray photograph without contrast medium (and not always then) can never show whether a fragment of disc is displaced or not, all sorts of radiological irrelevancies are adduced. In my experience, judges have learnt to ignore these false trails, but it would clearly save much time if they were recognised as such from the start and not put forward at all.

Evidence of spinal arthritis

Such evidence is to be expected; for few people reach middle age without the appearance of such X-ray evidence of wear and tear in one or other spinal joint. As age advances, bony outcrops called osteophytes develop at the edges of the vertebral bodies, gradually increasing in size as the years go by. At the neck, osteophytes usually form first at the fifth cervical level, spreading to adjacent vertebrae, and sometimes to all seven joints. If the patient has a considerable convexity at the back of the chest, bony spikes projecting forwards appear at the thoracic joints in early middle age. At the lumbar joints, the fourth and/or fifth are usually affected, but sometimes the third as well, or even alone. If the osteophytes are confined to the upper one or two lumbar vertebrae, the cause is usually one severe injury, often with slight permanent wedging of one vertebral body.

Evidence of spinal arthritis is often put forward to indicate that, quite soon, the patient would have developed pain in that area anyhow. Quite apart from the fact that the slow development of an osteophyte cannot cause pain coming on suddenly, this is a wholly misleading allegation. Spinal pain results from a displacement pinching sensitive tissue. This occurs in joints without, no less than those with, osteophytes. The outcrops themselves are irrelevant. Were this not so, almost every elderly person would be in permanent pain.

Once an osteophyte has formed, it can never get smaller, though it does, of course, tend to get larger as time goes on. Hence, if a patient is subject to attacks of pain, or had symptoms that in due course subsided, this is added evidence that a bony outcrop cannot be the cause.

Evidence of disc degeneration

Just as spinal osteophytosis is all but inevitable as age advances, so is X-ray evidence of narrowing of one or more disc spaces. The photograph shows two or more vertebrae to be closer together than at other levels. This is correctly attributed to degeneration of the disc, leading eventually to attrition of cartilage. But cartilage is a tissue devoid of nerves; hence, erosion of cartilage is a wholly painless phenomenon, unless, rarely, it becomes so extreme that the disc disappears completely, allowing bone to grind against bone. If, in addition to the narrowing, part of the disc becomes displaced, pain results, just as it would if the same displacement occurred in a joint with a disc of normal thickness. In other words, simple erosion without displacement causes no symptoms. The extreme case of this phenomenon is the aged patient who has slowly lost perhaps 50 mm (2 inches) in height. In such a case, the X-ray photograph may well show all five lumbar discs, each about 10 mm (0.4 inch) thick, to have become completely eroded. The vertebral bodies now lie virtually in contact; yet, as is well known, these veterans suffer no backache.

Evidence of fracture

Fractures of a vertebral body unite in three months, where-upon bone pain ceases. But violence sufficient to damage bone may well have damaged the adjacent disc, too, though the X-ray photograph cannot demonstrate the crack in the cartilage. If so, attacks of pain caused by recurrent displacement of the injured part of the disc may go on indefinitely, in spite of clear evidence that the bone is firmly united. Bone is a tissue containing blood and can, therefore, heal.

Evidence of osteochondritis (Schauermann)

This appears during adolescence and is commonest at the upper lumbar and lower thoracic vertebrae. Clinically, a rounded convexity is seen and felt, at which movement, particularly movement backwards, is somewhat restricted. Of itself, it causes no discomfort, but if a disc-lesion develops at a joint thus affected, the same symptoms result as would do so if osteochondritis were not present; the tendency to recurrence, however, is considerably enhanced.

Evidence of Schmorl's nodes

These appear in adolescence in patients who have worked hard precociously. The nucleus pulposus may very gradually erode bone at the centre of the vertebral body and carve itself out a cup-shaped hollow there. This event is very much commoner in farmers' than in city-dwellers' children. Though bone is a sentient structure containing nerves, the attrition is so slow that, in fact, no pain is set up. The result is that the nucleus lies in a fixed position and is less able to bulge in any direction, including backwards. Hence, the development of such a node is likely to diminish the centrifugal force that leads to disc-protrusion. However, these nodes are apt to form at the lower thoracic and upper three lumbar vertebrae, whereas nineteen out of twenty disc-lesions lie at the fourth or fifth joint.

Evidence of congenital abnormality

Minor congenital abnormality is of itself painless, otherwise
there would be symptoms from the time of birth. Quite
often, the fifth lumbar joint is joined to the sacrum by an
enlarged transverse process on one or both sides. This leads
to fixation of the lumbo-sacral joint and extra strain on the
fourth joint, radiologically normal, where a precocious disc-
lesion is apt to form. Spina bifida is a defect in the bony
arch that forms the hinder part of the vertebra, where there
is no joint, and has no significance in any one case. It can,
however, be argued that any congenital abnormality may
lead to asymmetry of that vertebra, so that it skews on
movement, straining the adjacent joint. This is, in fact, so,
and over twenty years ago (Gillespie, 1949) an investigation
showed that, in patients with such advanced lumbar disc
trouble that an operation had to be undertaken for removal
of the protrusion, an inborn structural abnormality of some
sort was four times more frequent than in a control series.

Evidence of spondylolisthesis

This is relevant. If one vertebra, nearly always the fourth
lumbar on the fifth, or the fifth on the sacrum, has become
displaced forwards, an unstable joint results. This may of
itself cause backache or pain down both legs, but the
symptoms are much more often the result of a disc-lesion
appearing at the weak joint. It behaves just like disc trouble
without spondylolisthesis, causing attacks of lumbago or uni-
lateral sciatica, and the onset is often before a patient reaches
twenty. The instability of the joint leads to enhanced
liability to recurrence.

Evidence of scoliosis

An S-shaped spine may be present at birth, but is much more
likely to develop in adolescence. The sideways curve is
accompanied by fixed rotation leading to prominence at the
back of the trunk of the ribs on the convex side. Once bone
growth ceases at the age of eighteen, no further change in the
shape of the bones can occur. If a patient's legs are not the

same length, a factitious scoliosis is seen when he stands. The pelvis tilts to the side of the short leg, forcing an obliquity on the lower lumbar joints, and the individual corrects this deviation by tilting the thoracic spine the other way.

A scoliosis is not of itself painful, but disc-lesions can occur in patients with, as well as without, scoliosis.

Evidence of lordosis

Lordosis is the name of a shape; it is not a disease. It means that the patient has a concave curve to his back. Nearly everyone has a lordosis at the neck and again at the lower lumbar joints. In some, it is greater than in others, but there is no such disease as "an excessive lordosis" predisposing to backache. Some individuals have a perfectly straight back, devoid of lordosis, which gives them an agreeable carriage; but they, too, develop disc protrusions.

Evidence of kyphosis

This means a convex curve of the backbone: the opposite of lordosis. Almost everyone has some convexity at the thoracic extent of the spine. Again, it is the name of a shape, not of a disease.

9

Schools of Thought in Manipulation

The question of spinal manipulation has remained vexed all this century. Strong views are held, not least by those who have no practical experience of this treatment. The result is heat and sound, but little light. This controversy is understandable enough, since different groups manipulate in different ways for different reasons. Such a situation is, however, no excuse for attitudes based on emotion, but calls instead for calm investigation.

Doctors are apt to manipulate the spine in a tentative way when other alternatives are lacking, rather than because a positive indication has emerged based on logical interpretation of the physical signs found present. Lay manipulators, by contrast, with cheerful dogmatism manipulate those who cross their threshold and adapt their statement of what is amiss to the treatment they are about to give. They have, therefore, invented a number of phrases (see Figure 9:1) that sound convincing enough to the public, but are unacceptable—and rightly so—to nearly all doctors. Indeed, Rees (1972) humorously described the chief requirement for a diagnosis in backache as "a sound knowledge of spelling". Confusion reigns, not least because there exist four schools of thought in spinal manipulation: osteopathy, chiropractice, bonesetting and the orthopaedic medical approach maintained for the past twenty-five years at St Thomas's Hospital in London.

Adhesions	Neuritis
Backstrain	Osteophytosis
Degenerate disc	Postural strain
Displaced hip	Pulled muscle
Displaced pelvis	Rotated facet joint
Displaced sacro-iliac joint	Sacro-iliac strain
Displaced vertebra	Sciatica
Facet binding	Scoliosis
Fibrositis	Spinal arthritis
Lordosis	Spondylosis
Lumbago	Sprung back
Lumbar osteoarthritis	Strained lumbar ligament
Lumbo-sacral strain	Strained lumbar muscle
Muscle spasm	Torn muscle
Narrowed disc	Twisted pelvis

FIGURE 9:1 THE VARIOUS NAMES UNDER WHICH A LUMBAR
DISC-LESION MASQUERADES
The word used depends on the person the patient visits, rather than on
evaluation of the physical signs found present

Osteopathy

This system of healing was originally based on the idea that
all disease resulted from spinal derangements. In 1874, Still—
the founder of osteopathy—enunciated the hypothesis that
displacement of one vertebra on another compressed the
relevant spinal artery, causing diminished blood-flow and
disease of any organ whose circulation had thus become impaired. Later, when it was made clear to him that any spinal
dislocation large enough to block the artery would give rise
to complete paralysis, if not instant death from rupture of
the aorta, he changed this "rule of the artery" to pressure on
a nerve, disease being now alleged to result from the cessation
of vital force transmitted to an organ along the nerve.

This idea has scarcely been modified since and was maintained by all the leading British osteopaths at the inquiry in
the House of Lords in 1935. Search in the latest edition of the
English Osteopathic Blue Book reveals only the slightest
withdrawal from this absolutism: for musculo-skeletal disorders are still regarded as "the most important factor in
disease." During the last decade, the programme of European

osteopathic congresses has continued to announce lectures on the place of osteopathy in gynaecology, in renal and in arterial disease. There has clearly been little modification of Still's original thesis, groundless though it is.

According to Still's osteopathic ideas, then, the correction of spinal displacements constitutes both prevention and cure of most non-spinal illness. Here lies the difference between medical manipulation—merely one method of treatment for a small number of very prevalent disorders—and osteopathy, which embraces manipulation not only for spinal conditions but all sorts of other diseases as well. It thus provides an alternative system of medicine, but the osteopaths—on whom the burden of disproof lies—have put forward no evidence that all recent medical research is mistaken, nor any cogent confirmation of the alternative hypothesis that they proffer. This universality has lingered on for a hundred years, since the days, in fact, when it did at least have a negatively justifiable basis. At that time, nearly all doctors' medicines were just as useless in the cure of disease as was osteopathy; hence, there was nothing in it. No one could make this contention today. But the panacea aspect of osteopathy presents the main obstacle to the acceptance of spinal manipulation.

The British osteopaths are the most conservative group of healers I have encountered; they continue to maintain concepts and to apply methods put forward when osteopathy was first invented as if they were unalterable. It is this rigidity of osteopathic dogma that leads its adherents into conflict with the medical profession. It is easy to see, however, how this notion is perpetuated. For example: an elderly man's headache is wrongly attributed by a doctor to high blood pressure, when it is in fact merely due to ligamentous contracture at the upper cervical joints with, as commonly happens, radiation of pain to the skull. Treatment for the blood pressure has no effect, but a lay manipulator cures the headache by manipulating the cervical joints. Another example is that of patients with root pain felt at the front of the trunk as the result of a thoracic disc-lesion, in whom a mistaken diagnosis of heart disease, kidney disease, chronic appendicitis, and so on, has been arrived at. In these cases, manipulation proves curative after all sorts of other treatments have failed. These diagnostic errors naturally lead the public to suppose that osteopaths *can* cure visceral disorders, and the lay manipulators' image is enhanced. They know no better than believe it too.

It is examples like these that give rise to the strong divergence of opinion between doctors and the public on the subject, for the doctor asks for scientific theory and evidence; whereas the public wants a cure, and will believe any hypothesis, however ill-founded, if treatment apparently based on it brings relief. Many doctors, myself included, regard this aspect of osteopathic dogma as wholly mistaken; for there can be no *one* cause of disease nor any *one* treatment. By contrast, many doctors regard the manipulative work of osteopaths as effective, provided they encounter the right sort of case. If osteopaths would limit their claim to the logical proposition that minor spinal displacements should be treated by manipulation, doctors' reproach against them would soon abate.

In Britain, osteopaths manipulate with the laudable intention of restoring full movement to any spinal joint at which they consider they can detect restricted mobility. They also try to relieve muscle spasm about the joint, since they regard it (on grounds obscure to doctors) as damaging to the joint and to distant structures as well. In fact, muscle spasm about a deranged joint does not hurt, and merely serves to guard the painful joint against damaging movement—it is a secondary phenomenon. If, as happens sooner or later to almost everyone, the joints of the neck have stiffened, the osteopath has to manipulate here, even though the client's only complaint is, say, lumbago. Until I understood their basic intention, I was at a loss to grasp how they could manipulate joints of the spine, sometimes with unfortunate results, so far away from where the actual trouble lay. This intention also serves to explain how they can maintain that their treatment is completed, though symptoms have not altered. Once the follower

K

of Still has satisfied himself that he has restored full movement to all the spinal joints, it is my experience that he considers that no more need be done.

There are believed to be fifty doctors in England practising
osteopathy.

The osteopathic lesion

This is defined by osteopaths as fixation of a spinal joint in
a faulty position within its range of movement without
irreversible change. Stoddard, the author of the standard
British book on osteopathy, states categorically that the osteopathic lesion is *not* synonymous with the disc-lesion. There is
no doubt that such fixation occurs, as merely looking at a
patient's back during acute lumbago immediately shows. The
lower back can be seen to be held bent forwards or sideways
and cannot be straightened (see Plate 1). Since 1947, succeed-
ing editions of my medical textbook have shown an X-ray
photograph of this deviation. Just as the knee becomes suddenly fixed in a faulty position within its range of movement
—that is, it cannot be straightened—when the cartilage in it
goes out of place, so can the same event show itself in the
same way at a spinal joint when a fragment of the cartilaginous disc becomes displaced. Alas, it is obvious that the "osteopathic lesion" is merely an evasive term for an ordinary
disc-lesion. The joint is held obliquely to make room for the
displaced fragment; this is the only mechanism whereby a
joint can suddenly become locked.

It was medical research that finally elucidated the nature of
the "osteopathic lesion." Dandy (1929) and Mixter and Barr
(1934) in the USA showed that sciatica could result from disc
protrusion. Lumbago was first attributed to the same lesion
(Cyriax, 1945) in England. Doctors, patients and osteopaths
were all agreed that a click during spinal manipulation often
signalled immediate recovery. X-ray photographs had already
shown that the bone did not shift. What other tissue exists that
is hard enough to click as it moves and is so placed as to jam
a joint? There is only one answer: a fragment of disc.

In fact, Still first advocated lumbar manipulation for putting a vertebra back. This idea was abandoned when X-ray photography showed that the bone had not moved. Then came the turn of the sacro-iliac joint, minor displacements of which could not be expected to show radiologically. Then the disc was accepted. Now, osteopaths are veering towards the facet joint becoming fixed (their term is "binding") but they have never explained how two smooth parallel surfaces are supposed suddenly to become fixed together (see Figure 9:2).

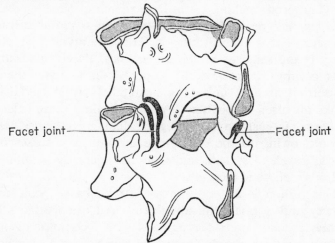

FIGURE 9:2 FACET JOINT

Osteopathy in the USA in Recent Years

The position of osteopathy in the USA was radically changed by the unexpected findings of a committee of medical men appointed by the American Medical Association in 1951 to study relations between osteopathy and medicine. Five doctors were chosen to decide whether or not osteopathy was still to be categorised as "cult healing". They reported in 1952, 1953 and finally in 1955, by when its members had visited six out of the seven schools of osteopathy in the country. The committee established that osteopathic teaching had long veered away from concentrating on manipulation. At their schools they were in the process of abandoning the "osteopathic lesion" thus showing themselves far in advance of their British counterparts by whom (even the medically qualified) it is still accepted today. In due course this logical expansion towards normal medical and surgical concepts would enable the graduates of osteopathic schools to achieve professional registration on a par with doctors. Already the public scarcely distinguished between them.

The gist of the reports follows: All schools of osteopathy are "non-profit making". The Department of Health subsidises teaching and research. The pre-registration requirements are the same as for medical schools. The time involved in clinical study is the same as at the universities. Purely medical subjects occupy 90 to 95% of students' time—again the same proportion as at a university hospital. Normal medical text books are used throughout. Actual teaching time, calculated in hours, is just on 25% higher than in ordinary medical schools, owing to the extra time devoted to diseases of the musculo-skeletal system, and their treatment by manipulation and other physical methods.

This tuition is an addition to that on basic medicine and surgery and normal clinical subjects. All osteopathic schools possess special clinics for patients with locomotor disorders. All osteopathic schools accept the normal medical views on disease and there has been no instance of adherence to Still's concept of a panacea. It is true that they do hold fast to the importance of musculo-skeletal lesions but do not maintain that correction of such lesions can cure organic disease.

The quality of training at medical schools is, on the whole, higher than at osteopathic, but the best of the osteopathic schools is better than the least satisfactory medical school. Tuition cannot therefore be regarded as sectarian or inadequate. Complete integration between medical and osteopathic schools can be envisaged and members of the American Medical Association may ethically accept posts in osteopathic schools.

This welcome change has had one unfortunate effect, however. As the osteopaths widened their horizons, both diagnostically and therapeutically, they increasingly abandoned manipulation. In consequence, the void that they had filled in their early days reappeared, now to become occupied by the next-comers in the cure-all business – chiropractors. Whereas osteopaths in the USA developed ever higher standards until they finally equalled doctors, the chiropractors have maintained their bigotry. They have instead developed more and better methods for trading in public gullibility and for augmenting their own incomes. Commercial advice on these lines is in fact included in chiropractic courses, as reported by Smith and by Le Riche.

Chiropractice

Whereas European osteopaths handle the spinal joints, searching for lack of mobility, chiropractors feel for vertebral displacements. Oddly enough, this puts them into the position of being the most direct followers of Still's original dictum. Chiropractice was modestly described in 1935 at the inquiry in the House of Lords as "the science of palpating and adjusting the articulations of the human spinal column by hand only." This is a perfectly acceptable statement, but recent chiropractic assertions no longer stop at that. I have in my possession a printed pamphlet issued a few years ago by chiropractors which even advises manipulation for the spots on the face known as acne, and a book written during the fifties in which typhoid fever and tuberculosis are listed as suited to chiropractice. Each thoracic vertebra is allocated to a different organ, except the sixth, which is called the "middle vertebra." How seriously does the author hope that such views can be taken? As recently as 1958, another chiropractor writing in his journal maintained that the fifth and sixth cervical vertebrae were out of joint in tonsillitis, the tenth thoracic vertebra in kidney disease and the second lumbar vertebra in constipation. In his view, this principle applied to all infectious disease. Remarkable figures, published by the Parker Chiropractic Research Foundation in the USA are quoted in R. L. Smith's critical review of chiropractice (*At your own Risk,* Trident Press, New York, 1969). They were reprinted in broadsheets advertising chiropractice delivered to householders in Melbourne and Sydney in 1970, and represent an analysis of a quarter of a million cases. The conditions treated include arthritis, diabetes, epilepsy, heart disease, high blood pressure, kidney and liver disorders, obesity, piles and ulcers. The lowest number of visits was twenty-two (for appendicitis!) and the greatest was eighty-four (for jaundice). It is scarcely credible that so considerable a number of patients proved gullible enough to submit to "treatment" by vertebral manipulation for such important illnesses, and equally remarkable that any body of healers exists prepared to carry it out. Chiropractors' excuse lies in stating (correctly) that all the tissues of the body possess nerves. Hence treating the nerves, which they falsely equate with "adjusting" the spinal joints, must have a universal effect. This is tantamount to averring that, because our lungs contain nerves, the treatment of pneumonia is not penicillin (which has saved millions of lives) but vertebral manipulation.

Many of osteopaths' manipulations are not very specific, being carried out by distant leverage and thus affecting several joints at a time. Chiropractors' manipulations are more exact and mostly consist of a thrust at one level. They make a speciality of manipulating the uppermost two joints of the neck—the only spinal joints that do not contain a disc—and there exists an extreme sect among them that regards manipulation of these two joints as enough for all purposes.

I am told that there are two doctors in England devoting themselves to chiropractice.

Bonesetting

This craft started centuries ago and continues now. The manipulators who call themselves bonesetters are largely persons who have an inborn flair for manipulation, or come from a family that has practised manipulation for generations.

The bonesetter does not set bones in the meaning of today —that is, reduce dislocations or fractures—but manipulates, alleging that he adjusts minor bony displacements only. He regards the click as a fragment of cartilage shifts, or the snap as an adhesion parts, as evidence that "the bone has been put back." This is not so, of course, as an X-ray photograph soon shows.

Bonesetters do not profess any cult; they have no theories on disease; they merely manipulate to the best of their ability those who come to visit them. There is a certain rough honesty here, even if their idea of what occurs is mistaken. I regard their infectious belief in their own powers as quite sincere.

Orthopaedic medical manipulation

To the orthopaedic physician manipulation for spinal trouble involves a series of passive movements manually performed. Anaesthesia is avoided. Before any manipulation is considered, clinical examination has had to show that the lesion is both spinal and suited to such treatment. Re-examination after each manoeuvre enables the effect to be accurately assessed. No endeavour is made to force full range at any spinal joint; once bony outcrops have formed in middle-age, this is impossible. The aim is pain-free movement at the joint, coupled with relief from symptoms. The two are not necessarily simultaneous; for example, where a patient with a cervical disc protrusion causing pain down the arm is examined at intervals, the return of full movement at the neck joint often precedes recovery from the pain down the arm by a month or two.

There are less than a dozen orthopaedic physicians (as distinct from orthopaedic surgeons) in the world—a world where patients are searching everywhere for an informed opinion on their spinal joints and, for that matter, on all the other moving parts of the body with which orthopaedic medicine deals. So insignificant a number can make no impact on the large mass of people seeking orthopaedic medical (as opposed to orthopaedic surgical) advice. It is this welter of patients which, despairing of finding an interested doctor, turns to all sorts of lay healers, not always in vain. I cannot see how any improvement can be expected until each orthopaedic department at every hospital in the country contains an orthopaedic physician working side by side with the orthopaedic surgeon in the same team. This is what was done at St Thomas's Hospital with the establishment of a happy collaboration, of great benefit to patients. Though in theory the surgeon could also do all the non-surgical work himself, he has his day filled with important duties to patients with severe injuries and diseases. However, the creation of a new division of medicine and new posts is extremely difficult, even if it is obvious that such a policy would save a nation ten or even a hundred times the outlay.

Medical work by lay manipulators

Britain is a free country—in some respects, too free. For example, it is not illegal for an ordinary person to perform a surgical operation or administer an anaesthetic agent. There is, equally, complete freedom for anyone at all to make a living by manipulation. Hence, any individual has a perfect right, without a day's tuition, to call himself an osteopath, to add the letters *DO* after his name, and to manipulate all comers as from that moment. In consequence, the British people, once they start searching for spinal manipulation, are compelled to go to anyone who chooses to apply the label to himself. Statistically, they are more apt to prove unlucky than lucky. Of the lay manipulators listed in the London telephone directory, only one-third have had even such training as enables them to be listed on the osteopaths' register. In other parts of Britain the proportion is probably lower still. This unfortunate situation clearly redounds to the public detriment, and a change whereby some guaranteed training had to be followed before a manipulator could start practising would be an advantage to all. In France, lay osteopathy is illegal and, since 1962, only registered medical practitioners have been allowed to manipulate. The arrangement in the USA is much sounder. There, an osteopath has to pass the same two pre-clinical examinations as do medical students, branching off only for the final period of training. Hence, there the prospective client knows that he is attending a practitioner who has followed an acceptable course of official tuition, leading to graduation by supervised examination.

10

Orthopaedic Medicine: the Problem and the Solution

Some doctors manipulate the spine often; they form a small minority. Most doctors manipulate never. Some employ anaesthesia; others, including myself, regard anaesthesia as dangerous. This confusion can be resolved only by the adoption of the same scientific detachment towards spinal troubles as is observed in dealing with other diseases. Most of the adverse opinions voiced today are based on the results of spinal manipulation carried out on manifestly (to a doctor) unsuitable cases or by people who do not know how to do it. Many doctors warn patients against visiting a lay manipulator; this is quite just, since the patient cannot distinguish the trained from the untrained. However, there is no reason to abhor manipulation when carried out by trained personnel under proper auspices. Unfortunately, facilities in this field in Britain remain so scarce that, as a result, most spinal manipulation is carried out by those who have never received any proper tuition.

Assessment of lay manipulators

There are no exact figures but, at the inquiry in the House of Lords in 1935, over two thousand people were believed to be making a living by manipulation. (Report from the Select Committee of the House of Lords Appointed to Consider the Registration and Regulation of Osteopaths Bill (HL) together with the Proceedings of the Committee and Minutes of Evidence, HMSO 1935.) There must have been a considerable increase since. If the figure is taken at three thousand now and is contrasted with the less-than-three-hundred appearing on the osteopaths' list, it becomes clear that a patient selecting a manipulator at random stands about one chance in ten of finding a trained operator.

Doctors' views on the safety and the results of spinal manipulation cannot fail to be coloured by what they see of the work of these lay manipulators, whose lack of medical training precludes their examining the patient properly. Many content themselves with running their fingers down the vertebrae and feeling the bones and joints for "displacements" or stiffness. This is followed by a standard spinal routine. No one working in this way could possibly tell whether a patient needed manipulation, let alone at what level to apply his treatment.

It can be argued, of course, that it is up to the patient who goes to a layman for manipulation to be sure that he needs it. The burden of diagnosis lies with the patient; the manipulator merely does what is asked of him. This is very much what usually happens in practice, but it does not seem at all likely that the potential client appreciates the position. In consequence, ludicrous errors are encountered —for example, manipulation of only the neck for sciatica. Serious errors are encountered, too, and later these have to be coped with by doctors, who again have their bias against manipulation reinforced.

An equally bad impression is created when patients with diseases entirely unconnected with the spine report long courses of fruitless manipulation by enthusiastic cultists. The fact that these people make all sorts of untenable claims for the results of spinal manipulation naturally evokes justified incredulity from the scientifically minded. If much of what a man says is unfounded, the tendency is to disbelieve the whole. In this instance, the analogy does not hold. Lay manipulators' theories may have little foundation, but their practice has many successes. Doctors must learn not to be put off spinal manipulation merely by weird statements of what is being attempted and why.

No one has made his calling more suspect to doctors than the lay manipulator. Nevertheless, his name stands high with many members of the public and he has prospered despite understandable lack of support from the medical profession.

Doctors' neglect

Medical men must learn to study not the failures of lay manipulators but their successes. Every family doctor knows of successful spinal manipulations carried out by a lay manipulator in patients previously treated without avail under the highest medical auspices. It has been customary to write these results off by assuming that such patients are neurotics, of which there is always a small number. By far the greater proportion, however, consists of responsible people, anxious to get well and back to work, who have bowed to their friends' insistence when it became evident that the medical profession had nothing effective to offer. This satisfied group, whatever the size in relation to the whole of those patients treated by lay manipulators, bears witness to neglect of a simple therapy. In my view, those medical men who do not countenance spinal manipulation under any circumstances are hardly less to blame than those lay manipulators who always try it on every client.

It is this neglect of spinal manipulation by the medical profession, coupled with the frequency of minor disc protrusions suitable for such manipulation, that has created the hiatus into which so many varieties of cultists have happily stepped. Our continued lack of interest, even after the way in which spinal manipulation achieves its good results had been scientifically elucidated, has enabled lay manipulators to establish themselves very cosily. The result is that doctors now find to their discomfort that they are virtually ousted from a field they once scorned to occupy. In London, at least, patients with backache often do not bother their doctor at all, but go straight to a lay manipulator. Alternatively, they do go to the doctor but ignore any warning he may give. Indeed, it is a waste of time, not to say inaccurate, to tell a patient, various of whose friends have been put right by this means, that it is a useless measure. This serves only to confirm the patient's previous opinion that doctors know little about, and possess an incomprehensible bias against, spinal manipulation. Philip Noel-Baker MP in a letter to *The Times* in 1963 criticised fruitless visits to doctors for a minor spinal displacement quickly put right by a lay manipulator. It must not be forgotten, however, that the successes are blazoned abroad; failures keep mum.

It is, however, not enough for doctors merely to point out that many of lay manipulators' claims are demonstrably false. This does not abate the public's confidence in, nor recourse to, them one whit. What doctors must do is to show patients that they are conversant with the uses and abuses of manipulation, and are as ready to prescribe it in suitable cases as to withhold it when contra-indicated. One important error in logic must be avoided—to abhor manipulation because of dislike for lay manipulators. The more a medical man dislikes manipulation by lay manipulators, the more trouble he should take to ensure that all those patients needing manipulation are sent at once to a medical colleague expert in this type of case, or to a physiotherapist trained in these methods. Unhappily, this is the very policy that is so rarely adopted, doctors' prejudice against lay manipulators often being extended to include manipulation itself. This absence of guidance forces the patient to go off to do the best he can on his own initiative.

Those of us who, understandably enough, dislike medical work being performed outside our sphere, must realise that the only way to obviate manipulation by lay manipulators is for our profession to investigate the uses of manipulation, reach agreed conclusions on indications for and against, and then employ it ourselves whenever necessary. We should also go beyond the techniques invented a century ago, and use methods superior to those of lay manipulators. A medical counter, based on scientific thought and evidence, would then at last balance the unfounded assertions of lay manipulators. Doctors approaching the problem with an open mind will find that the subject is perfectly straightforward; it has merely been clouded in the past by the obscurantist assertions of lay enthusiasts.

An important aspect of a changed attitude towards manipulation involves teaching. The family doctor soon gets to know of the successes of lay manipulators and the situation regarding manipulative treatment as it exists today is deplored by every one of them. But the patient is not attending hospital, and the consultant there probably never realises what happens. In consequence he, who alone is in a position to teach medical students, cannot draw their attention to the benefits of spinal manipulation. Medical students in general hear about this treatment only after they have graduated; by then, it is difficult for them to approach an entirely novel subject. Ignorance still exists, therefore, and remains self-perpetuating, running on into the time when the student himself becomes a consultant.

The solution

How can the present situation be rapidly changed for the better? It can in fact be done. There are two solutions:

1   Lay manipulators should put their house in order
     and receive State registration
2   The physiotherapists should take over

The first proposition I regard as impracticable in the UK; the second is what I have advocated ever since 1949, when my book, *Osteopathy and Manipulation,* appeared. It awaits only the goodwill of the Chartered Society of Physiotherapy.

In fact after years of pressure from myself their syllabus was amended in 1965 to include spinal manipulation. Unhappily, when the Society issued its revised syllabus in 1973, undergraduate tuition in manipulation was excluded. In order to mitigate the effects of this retrograde step, I offered to give weekend courses on the fundamentals of this work to all such final-year students as were interested. This suggestion was rejected.

Recognition of lay manipulators

Were these laymen to climb down and hold themselves out merely as practitioners of spinal manipulation, able and willing to treat patients sent to them for this purpose by medical men, recognition would follow in due course. Acceptance of this ethic would, in the long run, result in their receiving more patients. These would, moreover, be suffering from disorders suited to spinal manipulation.

The public would expect the same protection as is afforded by the examining boards of the medical profession and its auxiliaries: selection of subjects and supervision of the course of training by medical men; approved tuition at recognised hospitals; outside medically-qualified examiners. Graduates would receive State registration. Were this policy adopted, doctors could at last send patients requiring spinal manipulation confidently to trained and properly qualified medical auxiliaries. The speed of medical progress may well engender a favourable climate for this reform. Lay manipulators with foresight must be realising that the large advances that medical research has been and is now making must soon prove to all that osteopathy is not the panacea it used to be. However conservative they may be, those who regard spinal displacements as the common cause of all disease might consider themselves well-advised to step down gradually before events overtake them completely.

Factors militating against recognition

This reorientation would be wholly unacceptable to

British laymen, for the simple reason that they are very much better off carrying on as they are outside the medical sphere. The fees of lay manipulators in private practice often exceed those of the local doctors because the former are in such short supply. For years, one bonesetter in Cornwall had a waiting list of three months, although he saw a new patient each fifteen minutes. Acceptance of, say, a physiotherapist's salary and working within the National Health Service would spell financial hardship, which few might be prepared to undergo. Though, therefore, many complain to their patients that they are not "recognised" by the medical profession, it is in fact greatly to their benefit that they are not.

The other bar to reform is that doctors, held back by justified lack of confidence in the general run of lay manipulators, tend not to send patients requiring spinal manipulation to these people. They would like to send them to a hospital, but hospitals are ill-equipped to offer this treatment on a scale at all commensurate with the requirement. Once doctors were satisfied that lay manipulators were properly qualified for the work, their attitude would change. But the time-lag would be considerable, and these men have got to earn a living in the meantime.

Manipulation by physiotherapists

My principal solution (for details, see Cyriax 1949) is that the physiotherapists should take over. It was then, and remains now, the only immediately feasible proposition, and has been capable of implementation at any time during the last twenty years. It remains unrealised today, but I am still hoping for a change of heart.

As long as spinal manipulation remains a subject that arouses emotion, illogical attitudes will abound; the remedy is the adoption or avoidance of manipulation on rational grounds only. Such impartiality can scarcely be expected from a consultant whose department does not contain a trained manipulator, nor from those lay persons who earn their living purely by manipulation. But this is the very selectivity that evolves naturally in the doctor-physiotherapist team, provided that the physiotherapist is trained in manipulation. Between them they have every facility: informed selection of cases, a wide range of different types of treatment, alternative approaches when it is clear that manual methods cannot avail. There is everything to be said, therefore, for manipulation by physiotherapists, on the lines maintained at my hospital department over the last twenty-five years. The only immediately practicable solution is to ensure such tuition for all physiotherapy students. As they qualify, they will gradually fill the hospitals of Britain with skilled personnel. Within a few years, all physiotherapy departments would be able to offer manipulation to all those in need and the lay manipulators would become superfluous.

In my experience, physiotherapists have proved admirably suited to this work. They have a practical bent; they know their anatomy well (the standard they reach is scarcely below that of medical students); they learn the function and feel of joints and muscles; they study movement in all its branches; they develop strong, sensitive and apt hands; they have time and patience; they are accustomed to working with doctors and preserve a strict ethic towards them. Not only that, but they are the very people to whom patients needing manipulation have been sent for years, though unhappily all too seldom with the request for it.

Physiotherapists offer the further advantage that they are not indoctrinated with the ideas of one cult or another; they merely want to get the patient well as quickly as possible. If there are good manoeuvres in osteopathy, others in chiropractice, yet others in oscillatory techniques—they can use them all, whereas most lay manipulators regard it as apostasy to go outside the rigid framework of one sect. Eclectic manipulation, so that the measure best suited to any one lesion is selected, must be the medical aim.

It is important to realise that I have never taught manipulation in a vacuum, as an isolated craft. My students have not merely had to learn a series of manual techniques; I have

L

always insisted upon inculcating judgement at the same time. They have always been well-grounded in clinical examination, and in the indications and the contra-indications for manipulation. They know how to identify suitable and unsuitable lesions, how to apply safeguards and how to adapt technique to diagnosis.

Objections to manipulation by physiotherapists

A conservative attitude towards any advocacy of change is always to be expected from those whom it will inconvenience. The idea of manipulation by physiotherapists is no exception, though it would clearly benefit not only patients but physiotherapists themselves. Tuition to others involves the teacher learning it first, and there are forty schools of physiotherapy in Britain. At any time during the last twenty-five years, this would have meant the seconding of a teacher from each school to St Thomas's Hospital: the only school teaching physiotherapy students such methods. This scheme did not commend itself to the Society.

It has been argued that not all doctors wish physiotherapists to manipulate; this is true and will continue until all doctors are given the opportunity of seeing the physiotherapist prove her worth. Unanimity among medical men will never be attained. Ten years ago, a doctor in Hertfordshire sent a questionnaire to ninety-two family doctors (Wilson, 1962) and seventy-five answered "yes" to the question: "Is there a place for manipulation in orthodox practice?" If over three-quarters of all doctors are in favour of manipulation, sufficient majority surely exists to enable the Chartered Society of Physiotherapy to accept a policy of grounding all its students in manipulation.

It has been alleged that manipulation takes too long to learn. This is not so; the methods that I taught can be acquired in a few months. It is true that the osteopathic school in London takes four years to impart adequate knowledge of technique, but their manoeuvres are quite different. For this reason, my students have sometimes succeeded when experienced lay manipulators had already failed. In fact, manipulation cannot be difficult to learn; for most lay manipulators in Britain have had no tuition at all and yet possess satisfied clients. Nor can it be particularly dangerous, or these persons would find themselves repeatedly in the courts.

Some opposition is based merely on lack of experience of the essential service a manipulating physiotherapist offers to a hospital. But the real antagonists, understandably enough, consist of those who see their livelihood threatened. Lay manipulators everywhere naturally harbour the strongest dislike for my views and intentions. Indeed, we have it on the jubilant authority of the principal of the British School of Osteopathy that my efforts to transfer the public's confidence in manipulation from his members to physiotherapists has failed (*Medical News*, 5 February 1969). The repeated dramatic successes of lay manipulators have depended on even the simplest spinal manipulation remaining all but unobtainable by way of the medical profession for all these years. They have thus been able to create an aura of delicate touch and esoteric knowledge by using simple manual techniques. Their reputation stands high with many members of the public, and medical deprecation has had no effect, for the simple reason that no alternative has been offered. But mystique would soon evaporate if every doctor could order spinal manipulation for any patient, and it were then carried out in full view by a physiotherapist at the nearest hospital department.

Experience in other countries
Wherever physiotherapists trained at St Thomas's have travelled, their skill has commended them to doctors and patients. Eighteen years ago, my senior physiotherapist lectured and demonstrated in New Zealand, visiting every large hospital there, and manipulation by physiotherapists has been taken for granted in that country ever since.

Fifteen years ago, in Norway, a physiotherapist who had spent some months at St Thomas's began teaching groups of physiotherapists manipulation; he still does. These post-graduate students were examined by myself and the names of those who passed appear on a special list which doctors still consult when requesting such treatment. After two years, the health service there found recovery from some common disorders so much expedited that the physiotherapist's fee for a session of manipulation was voluntarily doubled.

Next came a report from Pringle in Dublin (1956) on the result of physiotherapists using the St Thomas's methods in acute lumbago: the time off work was halved.

Two other doctors, Troisier and Hirschfeld, each of whom started by employing a St Thomas's graduate, reported similar experiences from Paris and Bremen.

Two physiotherapists, Kaltenborn in Norway and the other in Australia, have both adopted my methods of assessing the lesion by clinical examination, but manipulate in ways different from each other and from me. But, in each case, proper selection of patients is assured. For the last six years, all physiotherapy students in Norway have learnt and been examined in manipulative techniques; in Australia (Adelaide), the same applies at the school where the Vice-Principal is a St Thomas's graduate. In Canada, when the move to teach all physiotherapy students vertebral manipulation was put forward, the chiropractors in Ontario were so alarmed that they filed a petition to the Minister of Health there to prohibit physiotherapists manipulating (August, 1974). This plea indeed provides a sincere tribute to trained physiotherapists' competence in this field. They employ methods with no resemblance to chiropractice, as anyone glancing at my book for them can see.

I mention all these facts to emphasise that I am not alone in regarding manipulation by physiotherapists as welcomed by medical men and patients.

11

Argument for a New Establishment

At this moment, thousands of people are in pain and off work with, amongst other disorders of the moving parts, a slipped disc. This is so, not because the way to put it right is unknown, but because there are far too few physiotherapists trained in manipulation and too few orthopaedic physicians to go round. Hence, even a method devised more than two thousand years ago, and well-known today by doctors and patients to be effective, cannot reach those who need it. Doctors' interest in the non-surgical aspect of orthopaedics has proved difficult to arouse. My extension to physiotherapists of tuition on the indications for, and technique of, manipulation has encountered strong resistance from their leaders for years. Here then is a vast hiatus, now filled largely by lay manipulators. There is no other branch of medicine in which the patient is forced to frequent irregular practitioners for sheer lack of medical, or medically trained, personnel. After all, there are no diabeticopaths, cardiopractors or nerve-setters. Though they do not know it, these sufferers are all seeking an orthopaedic physician. But, understandably enough, they have never heard of such a doctor, and so have to do the best they can with whoever offers. Some derive satisfaction, others not, from lay manipulators, bone-setters, acupuncturists, faith-healers, nature-curers, or "the waters."

Everyone suffers at intervals throughout his life from the disorders with which orthopaedic medicine deals. Sooner or later, we sprain our knee or ankle, hurt our back, crick our neck, strain our shoulder or elbow, or develop sciatica. These disorders collectively account for more invalidism than any other types of trouble, and they happen to be among the easiest to relieve. All that is needed is enough doctors and physiotherapists trained in this discipline to staff hospitals everywhere. Patients would soon flock to them and the problem would be solved. In my view, attached to every orthopaedic team in the world should be an orthopaedic physician working daily with the orthopaedic surgeon. The same collaboration would then be created as now exists between neurologist and neurosurgeon, gastro-enterologist and abdominal surgeon. Such a colleague would relieve the orthopaedic surgeon of the very work he enjoys least—the non-surgical aspect of diseases of the moving parts.

The fact that no post in orthopaedic medicine is offered at any hospital anywhere has, of course, had a strong deterrent effect on the actual recruitment of young doctors tentatively drawn towards this speciality. Applicants for training for a non-existent job have naturally not proved numerous, however vital their existence may be to the working capacity of the community. Here lies the main reason for the lack of appeal that orthopaedic medicine makes, though this is the tuition that I offered continuously for thirty years, until my retirement from St Thomas's Hospital in 1969.

This hiatus costs untold sums in avoidable invalidism. Who would ever have supposed that in Britain, for instance, the main losers—the Confederation of British Industry, the Department of Health and Social Security and the Insurance Companies—would, between them, have proved impotent to relieve themselves of a huge financial burden by enjoining the creation of an institute of orthopaedic medicine on the lines started by Hirschfeld in Germany?

An institute of orthopaedic medicine

It is a remarkable fact that the medical man who wants detailed instruction in how to examine the moving parts of the body, what inferences can be drawn, and what treatment to prescribe has virtually nowhere to go in any country in the world. It is scarcely less remarkable that the doctor or physiotherapist who wants to learn when, when not, and how, to manipulate has really nowhere to go, either. The osteopaths offer a two-year course to state-registered physiotherapists and a nine-month course to doctors, but in both instances those taking the courses become embroiled in manipulation as a near-panacea, in theories about the osteopathic lesion, the cure of diseases not connected with the spine, and so on. Moreover, they are taught the manoeuvres based on Still's century-old notion of the displaced vertebra rather than those designed to shift a fragment of disc. By contrast, orthopaedic medicine embraces the whole body, not just the spine, and manipulation forms only a small part of the effective treatments employed.

If just one institute of orthopaedic medicine existed in each country in the world, patients requiring this approach would have somewhere to go. Doctors would have a centre where the methods of examination and treatment would be on view and taught daily throughout the year. Physiotherapists wishing for a grounding in these methods would also be welcome. At any time during the last twenty years, the situation could have been resolved in this way and the present plethora of manipulating laymen gradually rendered superfluous. Such an institute would have regained for medicine a field that was, by default, relegated to unsatisfactory personnel.

Reversal of policy on physiotherapy

It is a sad paradox that my years of advocacy of manipulation by doctors and physiotherapists have had the reverse effect of that intended. Dissemination of my views has led patients to demand manipulation more and more overtly, doctors to offer diminishing resistance to so logical a proposition, and patients in the absence of an alternative to frequent lay manipulators ever more confidently. Did they but know it, the leaders of the Chartered Society of Physiotherapists in Britain have held lay manipulators in the hollow of their hand for the last twenty years. These men have reason to be extremely grateful to the Society's teachers. So far, their policy of withholding instruction on manipulation from their students has served only to maintain the near monopoly, and thus the prosperity, of lay manipulators at the expense of graduates of their own society. It has not thereby even ingratiated itself with medical men; for, in the main, they want physiotherapists to manipulate. Immediate reversal of this negativism, coupled with the use of such teachers and examiners as now exist, might still swing doctors and the public round to the physiotherapists' side, though every year of further delay makes such a change of attitude more difficult. Unfortunately the Society's latest move has been a retrograde step. Their new syllabus, promulgated in 1973, subsitutes mobilising techniques for the previous manipulation, thus resoring laymen's ascendancy. If wholly untalented individuals can manipulate profitably, what is the matter with the trained physiotherapist? It has always been a mystery to me why the Society has been at such pains to help the ostesopaths at the expense of doctors and of its own members.

Over the years, lay manipulators have watched my endeavours with scorn—not without reason; for these efforts have so far got the practising physiotherapist nowhere. But it seems to me that attitudes are beginning to change and that this book may fall on less barren ground than the one I wrote for the general public in 1949.   Time will show.

Appendix

Car Seat Ratings
by Dr Bernard Watkin

Modern living entails an enormous amount of time spent sitting. For example, driving, office work, public transport of all forms, watching television, going to the theatre and cinema—all combine to make the day's activity into one of continuous sitting.

The effect of sitting (a fundamentally unnatural position) on the soft tissues of the spine has been explained in this book. Despite evidence of such effects, not much has been done by car manufacturers to design vehicle seats with adequate lumbar support and related seat cushion shape.

Where office and industrial seating is concerned, some British firms such as Tan-Sad, Sankey Sheldon and Conran-Ryman had made some progress. The designs of the Chair Company Limited of London are the most advanced ortho-paedically in the domestic and office range, with a pleasant non-medical appearance.

The star rating given to car seats takes the following criteria into account:

1   *Seat cushion:*
   (*a*) Degree of firmness
   (*b*) Thigh depth
   (*c*) Shape in relation to seat back
   (*d*) Height from floor

2   *Seat back:*
  (*a*) Degree of firmness
  (*b*) Amount of lumbar support provided
  (*c*) Correct shape elsewhere, including angle

The well-designed seat, in orthopaedic terms, should provide the appropriate shape, accompanied by sufficient firmness, to support the body correctly throughout the required range of postures. For example, the seat should combine lumbar support with thigh support without inhibiting circulation.

A head rest or neck restrainer should be an essential feature of a vehicle seat, minimising whiplash injury to the neck region on sudden deceleration or impact. They are now compulsory in the US, but are not included in this assessment because they are not, as yet, consistently provided in Europe.

The star rating is extremely concise. In theory it is a five-star scale, but in practice there is as yet no seat that justifies five stars—in other words, satisfactorily fulfils all the specified requirements. The three best seats have been given four stars, but they are still far from ideal.

Such a simplified system, with a flattened scale of ratings, inevitably obscures small points of difference between seats. Readers' personal preferences may well point in other directions. But the rating is intended as a convenient overall assessment based on specific criteria, for use as a quick guide by the purchaser. The star ratings may be interpreted as follows:
  *   *Bad*: could be orthopaedically harmful
  **   *Poor*: designed without taking orthopaedic considerations into account
  ***   *Moderate*: though still with inadequate support at certain points
  ****   *Adequate*: but capable of further development
  *****   Fulfils orthopaedic requirements well

Ratings as awarded did not take into account the amount of perspiration generally retained by modern upholstery. Some manufacturers—not only of luxury cars—are now introducing non-plastic porous fabrics.

Some seventeen makes of separate back rest are available, but only one provides adequate lumbar support. This is the Posture Curve, patented in Britain, the USA and Canada, which is suitable for domestic, car and office use. Details are obtainable from: F. Ashton Ltd., 16 Groton Rd., London SW18.

The conclusions of the rating are clear enough. Buying a luxury car provides no guarantee that adequate attention has been given to seat design. US car seats, on the whole, are the least suited to the human back. Volvo's high reputation is reasonably well justified. Very good seats were found in one Alfa Romeo model and the new Triumph Stag. Possibly the best—certainly the least complicated—of all is in the new Range Rover. This simple construction was advocated (by me) some years ago.

This assessment was made on models available for testing in December 1973.

MAKE AND MODEL	RATING	COMMENT
Alfa Romeo		
Guilia	**	
1750 GTV	****	One of the best tested
2000 GTV	****	Good, but surprised no development since 1972
Sud	***_	
American Motors		
Rambler	*	
Aston Martin		
V8	***	
Audi-NSU		
Audi 80	**	
Ro 80	**	
Austin		
Allegro SS	*+	
Alegro Special	*+	
Mini	*	
Mini Clubman	*+	Almost merits two stars
1100	*	
1300 GT	**	
1800	**	
Maxi	**	
Taxi cab (drivers seat)	*	Considering fatigue factors involved this is a very poorly designed seat
Bentley		
T-series	***	
BMW		
2002	**	
2002 Touring	*+	Disappointing compared with other BMW's
2500	***	
3.0 C.S.I.	***	Reasonable seat
3.0 C.S.L.	**_	
	****+	(BMW offer as an optional extra a well designed seat which is the best seat tested)
Buick	*	Comment on US Cars in general: very poor and well below European seating standards
Bristol	*	
Cadillac		
Eldorado	*	
Fleetwood Brougham	*	
Chevrolet		
Corvet 2 Rotor	*_	
Chrysler		
Hillman Avenger	*	
Hillman Avenger Super	*	

MAKE AND MODEL	RATING	COMMENT
Hillman Avenger GL	**−	
Hillman Hunter	**	
Hillman Hunter GL Est.	*	
Hillman Imp	**	
Hillman Imp Super	**	
Humber Sceptre	**	
Citroen		
DS 23	**	
GS 1220 Comfort Est.	**	
D Super 5	**	
Dyane 6	*−	
Daf		
33	**	
44	**	
55	**	
66	**	
66 Marathon	**	
Datsun		
1207 (Sunny)	*	
200 B (Bluebird)	*+	
Daimler		
Limousine (chauffeur seat)	*+	
Limousine (passengers seat	*+	
Sovereign (see Jaguar XJ6)		
Dodge		
Valiant	*	
Ferrari		
2+2	**++	
365 T (Berlinetta)	**−	
Dino	*+	
Fiat		
124	**+	
Automatic 132 Spec	**−	
Automatic 132 Sal	**−	
Automatic 127	**+	
Ford (*British*)		
Capri	**	
Consul 2000	**−	Too soft
Cortina	**	
Escort 1100 L	**++	Almost merits 3 stars
Granada	**−	Too soft
Ford (*American*)		
Continental MK IV	*	
Cougar XR7	*	
Mustang 11 Ghia	*+	
Ford (*Australian*)		
Fairmont	*−	

MAKE AND MODEL	RATING	COMMENT
Jaguar		
XJ 12 and 6	***_	
E-type	**	
Jensen		
Healey	**_	
Interceptor	***	
Lamborghini		
Countach	*_	Dreadful hammock type seat
Lancia		
Beta	***	
Lotus		
Elan	**	
Maserati		
Merak	**_	
Mercedes		
230	**	
450 SL	**	
280 SE	**	
MG		
MGB	*+	In keeping with sports car discomfort
Morgan		
4/4 1600	*	
+8	**+	
Morris		
Marina TC	*+	
Marina Est	*+	
Maxi HL	*+	Cloth seats
Moskovitch		
412 SAL	**	
Oldsmobile	**	
Opel		
Rekord	***	
Commodore	***	
Panther		
42	**+	
Peugeot		
104	*+	
404A	**	
504	**	Too soft
Plymouth	*	
Pontiac	*	
Porsche		
911 Targa 2.7	***++	
914	*_	

MAKE AND MODEL	RATING	COMMENT
Reliant		
Rebel	**	
Scimiter	**	
Renault		
4	**_	
5	**+	
6	**_	Too soft
12 TL	**_	Too soft
12 TS	***	Lumbar support incorrect —seat with potential for improvement
15 TS	**_	
16 TL	**_	Various shapes, all too soft
Rolls-Royce		
Corniche	***_	Too soft and bulky—waste of padding
Silver Shadow	***	
Rover		
2200	**	Overrated seating by salesmen
2200 TC	***_	Lumber support too low
3500	***_	Marginally better than 2200
Range Rover	****	Surprised this has not been developed further
Saab		
95	**	
Skoda		
S110 LS	**_	
S110 R Coupe	**+	
Simca		
1301 SAL. Spec	*+	
1100 LS	*	
1000 Spec	*	
1501 Spec	*	
Toyota		
1600 SAL deluxe	**	
1600 TS (or ST)	**+	
Corona	**	
Crown 2000 Est	**_	
Triumph		
Dolomite Sprint	**_	
GT6	***_	
1500 TC	***_	
Spitfire	***_	
Stag	****	Firmer than Dolomite tested. Lumbar support capable of improvement

TR6	**	
2000	**	
2.5 P.I.	**	
Vanden Plas		
1300 Princess	*+	
Vauxhall		
Magnum 2300	***	
Viva S.L.	***	Greatly improved range of
Ventora	***	seating. Lumbar support not
VX/90	***	yet correct
Viva Standard	**	
Viva Deluxe	**	
Volkswagen		
1200	**	
411 E	***	
LS Variant	***	
Passat	**+	
Beetle 1303 S	**	
Volvo		
144 E	***	Overrated seating by salesmen,
164 TE	***	spoilt by seat cushion shape.
		Not as good as older models
Wartburg		
Knight	**_	
Wolseley		
(See Austin 1800)		

Glossary

ACROPARAESTHESIA. Pins and needles in both hands.

ARTHRODESIS. Operative fixation of a joint leading to bony fusion.

BONESETTER. Old-time rustic manipulator who alleged that his manoeuvres "put a little bone back in place" when a click was heard.

BRACHIAL. Connected with the arm.

BRACHIAL NEURITIS. Pain in the arm and forearm due to pressure on a nerve root.

CARTILAGE. Gristle.

CHRONIC. Long-standing.

CEREBRO-SPINAL FLUID. The liquid enclosed by the dura mater in which the brain and spinal cord float—a shock-absorbing device.

CERVICAL. Connected with the neck. There are seven cervical vertebrae between the skull and the first thoracic bone.

CHEMONUCLEOLYSIS. Attrition of disc by action of enzyme (chyinopapain).

CONTRACTURE. Permanent shortening.

CONGENITAL. Present at birth, inborn.

DISC, INTERVERTEBRAL. The circular buffer lying between two vertebrae. It consists of a tough cartilaginous rim surrounding a soft nucleus.

DURA MATER. The membrane covering brain and spinal cord containing liquid in which they float.

EXTENSION OF TRUNK. Bending backwards.

FACET JOINT. A little joint at each side of the vertebra, formed by a downward projection from one bone which slides along an upward projection from the bone below.

FIBROSITIS. Strictly speaking, inflammation of fibrous tissue. Often used in the past as a misnomer for a minor disc displacement.

FLEXION OF TRUNK. Bending forwards.

FORAMEN (between two vertebrae). Circular opening through which the nerve root emerges.

HERNIA. Displacement from a cavity outwards.

KYPHOSIS. Convexity of spine.

LESION. Any deviation from the normal.

LIGAMENT. Strong fibrous band joining two bones.

LORDOSIS. Spinal concavity.

LUMBAGO. Sudden severe backache with temporary fixation.

LUMBAR. Connected with the lower back.

MANIPULATION. Treatment by movement carried out manually.

MANUAL. Connected with the hand.

MENISCUS. The cartilage lying between two bones, for example, at the knee.

MYELOGRAM. Photograph by X-rays of flow of opaque oil introduced into spinal fluid.

NERVE ROOT. The extent of a nerve where it emerges from the dura mater and traverses the gap between two vertebrae.

NEURASTHENIA. Undue emotional tension.

NEURITIS. Inflammation of degeneration of a nerve.

OSTEOCHONDRITIS OF SPINE. Adolescent wedging of vertebral body leading to localised convexity.

OSTEOPHYTE. Bony outcrop at the edge of a bone close to a joint.

PRONE. Lying face-downwards.

PROPHYLAXIS. Preventive measure.

REDUCTION. Putting back into proper position.

REFERENCE OF PAIN. Radiation of pain whereby it is

felt at a distance from its actual source—a misleading phenomenon.

SCAPULA. Shoulder-blade.

SCIATICA. Pain felt in the region of the sciatic nerve, i.e. in the buttock, back of thigh and calf.

SCHMORL'S NODE. A cavity at the centre of the vertebral body caused by the disc pressing vertically.

SCOLIOSIS. Sideways deviation of the spinal column.

SPINA BIFIDA. Inborn defect in bony arch of vertebra.

SPONDYLITIS. Inflammation of the spine.

SPONDYLOLISTHESIS. Slipping forwards of a vertebra on the one below.

SPONDYLOSIS. Thinning of an intervertebral disc and/or the existence of bony outcrops at the edge of the vertebra.

SUPINE. Lying face-upwards.

THERAPEUTIC. Effective as treatment.

THORACIC. Connected with the chest. There are twelve thoracic vertebrae, lying between the neck and lower back.

TORTICOLLIS, ACUTE. Sudden painful fixation of the neck in an abnormal position.

TRACTION. Pulling apart.

TRAUMATIC. Caused by injury.

VERTEBRA. The single bony segment, twenty-four of which form the spinal column.

References

Barbor, R. (1955), "Low backache", *Brit. med. J.* (*8 October*)

Browse, N. L. (1965), *Physiology and Pathology of Bed-Rest* (Springfield, Ill.: Thomas)

Brügger, A. (1960), "Documenta Geigy", *Acta rheumat., 18*

Collis, J. S. (1963), *Lumbar Discography* (Springfield, Ill.: Thomas)

Cyriax, J. (1945), "Lumbago", *Lancet, 2,* 427

Cyriax, J. (1948), "Fibrositis", *Brit. med. J., 2,* 251

Cyriax, J. (1949), *Osteopathy and Manipulation* (London: Crosby Lockwood)

Cyriax, J. (1950), "Treatment of lumbar disc-lesions", *Brit. med. J., 2,* 1434

Cyriax, J. (1970), *Textbook of Orthopaedic Medicine, 1,* fifth edition (London: Baillière, Tindall; Baltimore, USA: Williams & Wilkins)

Cyriax, J. (1975), *Textbook of Orthopaedic Medicine, 2,* ninth edition (London: Baillière, Tindall); Baltimore, USA: Williams & Wilkins)

Dandy, W. E. (1929), "Loose cartilage from intervertebral disc simulating tumour of spinal cord", *Arch. Surg., 19,* 660

Gillespie, H. (1949), "The significance of congenital lumbo-sacral abnormalities", *Brit. J. Radiol., 22,* 257, 270

Glorieux, P. (1937), *La Hernie postérieure du ménisque inter-vertébral* (Paris: Masson)

Gowers, W. (1904), "Lumbago", *Brit. med, J., 1,* 117

Hult, L. (1954), *The Munkfors Investigation* (Copenhagen: Munksgaard)

Mixter, W. J. & Barr, J. S. (1934), "Rupture of intervertebral disc", *New England J. Med., 211,* 210

Nachemson, A. (1959), "Measurement of intradiscal pressure", *Acta orthop. Scand., 28,* 269

Noel-Baker, P. (1963), Letter to *The Times* (5 February)

Pringle, B. (1956), "Approach to intervertebral disc-lesions", *Trans. indust. med. Offrs, 5,* 127

Rees, W. E. S. (1971), "Multiple bilateral subcutaneous rhizolysis of segmental nerves for intervertebral disc syndrome", *Ann. gen. Pract., 16,* 126

Sair Back (1967), "Symposium on clinical problems", *J. Coll. gen. Practit., 13,* 60

Sicard, A. (1901), "Les injections extradurales par voie sacrococcygienne", *C. R. Soc. Biol., 53,* 396

Smith, L. (1969), "Chemonucleolysis", *Clin. Orthop., 67,* 72

Index